#emphatic

#emend

#emprise

#employer

#employ

#embody

#empower

#emanate

#emotive

#embosom

#emollient

#eminence

#empoison

#embitter

#emotion

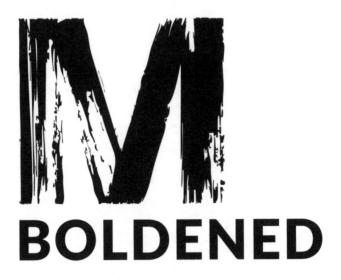

BOLDENED

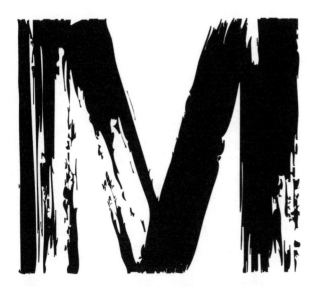

BOLDENED

MENOPAUSE CONVERSATIONS WE ALL NEED TO HAVE

EDITED BY CAROLINE HARRIS

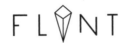

First published 2020

FLINT is an imprint of The History Press
97 St George's Place, Cheltenham,
Gloucestershire, GL50 3QB
www.flintbooks.co.uk

General Editor: Caroline Harris
Consultant Editor: Jo de Vries

British Library Cataloguing in Publication Data.
A catalogue record for this book is available from the British Library.

ISBN 978 0 7509 9406 4

Typesetting and origination by The History Press
Printed and bound in Great Britain by TJ Books Limited

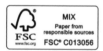

MIX
Paper from
responsible sources
FSC
www.fsc.org   FSC® C013056

Contents

Praise for *M-Boldened*

'Please read this book. It will save your sanity, enlighten you, support you and, I hope, make your menopause days sunnier.'

Kirsty Wark FRSE, award-winning BBC journalist and *Newsnight* **presenter**

♀

'It's thanks to women and conversations like these that the story of menopause as something to dread and suffer is changing to something to embrace and thrive through.'

Clare McKenna, acclaimed Irish radio and TV presenter and broadcaster

♀

'A powerful book that captures some raw truths and unique stories of menopause from woman across the globe. Thank you to Caroline Harris for her outstanding work on producing *M-Boldened*, a must read and a book that has the power to both unite and empower woman of all generations.'

Australian Nursing and Midwifery Federation

♀

'Menopause is a natural process to ageing but unfortunately due to cultural barriers many women in the traditional societies hide this change. On top of that due to a lesser focus on women's own health, a large number of women have no knowledge about the effects of menopause on their emotions and health. I hope this scholarship will be a great effort to help women to get answers to unsolved questions.'

Rukhshanda Naz, the first woman Ombudsperson-KP for the Protection of Women against Harassment at Workplace, activist and lawyer, previously Head of UN Women Pakistan's Khyber-Pakhtunkhwa/Federally Administered Tribal Areas division

♀

'This is a book that every woman needs to read. Unabashedly truthful and real. I'm so happy this discussion has finally started!'

Laura Dowling BSc(Pharm) MPSI, The Fabulous Pharmacist (@fabulouspharmacist)

♀

'The subject of menopause is very serious because this natural state which is part of the normal sexual and reproductive life of women is often negatively treated by harmful traditional behaviors [sic]. Postmenopausal women are thus excluded from sexual relations, including with their husbands, on the grounds that it would cause illnesses in them. One of the consequences of this practice is that all pathological bleeding, including that caused by cancer of the uterus, is paradoxically welcomed by victims who believe they are having a return to menstruation. In my long struggle against female genital mutilation, child marriage, and other harmful traditional practices, I have always spoken out against the harmful traditional practices including those associated with menopause. This is why I am very happy to see that renowned and very committed specialists like yourself [in reference to Dr Eleanor Nwadinobi, see Chapter 14] have participated in the in-depth analysis of the phenomenon of menopause through this excellent book entitled: *M-Boldened: Menopause Conversations We All Need To Have*, edited by Caroline Harris.'

Dr Morissanda Kouyaté, Executive Director of Inter-African Committee on Traditional Practices; laureate of the 2020 United Nations Nelson Rolihlahla Mandela Prize

♀

Beginning to Break the Silence

Strangely, I can't remember what age I was when my periods started, but I do remember the emotion that accompanied them: rage.

Rage at this uncalled-for transformation of my body. Rage at the lack of control; that I was no longer the person I had become accustomed to being; the remoulding of what and who I was and how I would be seen. Rage that I might bleed at any time (my periods were irregular for the first few years); that I would be 'caught out'. Rage, too, at becoming a woman – something that, from what I had picked up during childhood and early teens, and parts of my own family history, seemed a limiting, perhaps even dangerous, thing to be.

At the other end of my oestrogen lifespan, in 2015, rage was again my overriding and defining emotion. I was outraged not so much by the hot flushes (I used to suffer from chronic panic attacks, which for me were a considerably more horrible experience); not so much by the grief of my fertility ending (I had miscarried trying for a second child some years before and so had already faced losing my reproductive ability). It was more about the sensuality and embodiment of menopause: about sex, arousal, the forest architecture of my vagina and, particularly, how I smelled.

This may sound trivial, especially to those whose experience of menopause has been much more physically and psychologically challenging than mine, but for me, it struck at the heart of those feelings of lost control and of my body suddenly becoming another country. My geography – my ecosystem – was changing, and I was a stranger to myself in this strange land. I no longer got wet with desire when I expected to. My scent, when I explored, was not the soft fragrance I had known; instead, as I grappled with trying to pin down and name it, all I could think of was bitter seaweed and burnt rubber. Before menopause, my body was my 'familiar' and I felt comfortable with it, even in its ageing (well, most of the time, anyway). I had adapted to the changes that come after giving birth, and the anxieties that those transformations can bring. But this was something else. Somewhere else. And I didn't like it.

As I navigated through the physiological upheavals – like many others on the same journey, gathering information via the internet, and the occasional conversation with one or two friends – I was gripped by a different kind of anger. Why wasn't any of this being talked about? Why had I arrived at menopause so unprepared? Why had I not previously been made aware of any symptoms apart from hot flushes? The rhetoric of menopause seemed to be either silence or joke. And as much as humour can be essential in weathering both the absurdities of life and the particular difficulties we each face, all too often the 'jokification' of menopause is belittling, uncomfortable and barbed.

As I looked further, I began to unearth books and articles, from the feminist-inspired *Our Bodies, Ourselves* series, which arose from the Boston Women's Health Collective in the 1970s with its aims of empowering women through increased health awareness, to Gail Sheehy's *The Silent Passage*, first published in the early 1990s. In the original *Vanity Fair* article that laid the ground for her book, Sheehy referred to menopause as 'the last taboo, the stigma of stigmas'. This was more than twenty-five years ago; so why does it still feel bold and exposing to speak up publicly about menopause? Why can it still feel for so many of us as though we are making our way through this transition on our own, when it is something that will affect half the world's population who attain this stage of their lives?

I wanted to explore these questions: about what menopause is, and what it means not only individually, but in our wider societies. I wanted to hear from other people about their own experiences, knowledge and understandings, not only from my own position in the UK, but globally.

What is menopause?

The word 'menopause' is a relatively recent term, but in these times of cultural globalisation and tech-speak, it has established itself as the modern way to refer to this life transition. Coming from the ancient Greek via Latin, 'meno' means 'month' and through this the menses: women's 'monthlies' or periods; 'pause' is here an 'end' or 'stop', rather than a brief interlude. As a medical term, menopause was coined by a French doctor in 1821, according to sociologist Cécile Charlap, author of *La Fabrique de la Ménopause* (which can be translated as *The Construction of the Menopause*). From here it passed into the English language through the dialogue of nineteenth-century doctors discussing their surgical experiments on women (Emily Steinberg's 'Men O Pause' chapter, which relates some of this history, is a graphic account in more than one sense). 'Menopause' was first used in print in 1872 and became increasingly common during the twentieth century. Charlap notes that 'climacteric', more common today in the US, has a much longer history in this context: 'Inherited from antiquity, [it] was used to qualify this critical turning point in human ageing, thus not at all specific to women nor focused on the end of menstruation and fertility,' she explained in an interview with Sandrine Hagège for the French National Centre for Scientific Research (CNRS). 'The change' – the phrase my mother used to speak of her midlife in the late 1970s – today has mixed connotations; it may be seen as outmoded and related to old-fashioned ideas and stereotypes, and thus derogatory, but at the same time can offer a non-medicalised way of talking about transition.

Most people in the twenty-first-century West are used to viewing menopause through the lens of medical categorisations and processes: a language of symptoms, diagnoses, deficiencies, treatments, replacements. We list those we have, those we don't. Those we've tried, those we won't. Such naming can be an important step in understanding. Even after some years of regular panic attacks, for example, I still had no word for these profound bodily and emotional episodes. I vividly recall browsing the shelves of a a bookshop and first discovering a book that gave this daily scourging phenomenon a name. The panics immediately became more knowable, less scary. Symptom names can give us ways to define intense experiences of pain or amorphous senses of unease; ways to compare what we are going through with other people; courses of action we might therefore follow. But the medical language of menopause is not a friendly or attractive one; it is a lexicon of atrophy and dysfunction, of parts shrivelling, drying, not working according to the manual, and of offputting and impersonal drug and treatment names.

What if we enacted a new language, or a reclamation – as in the refiguring of 'queer' and 'crip'? Cat Chong (Chapter 11) brings our attention to the language around menopause and endometriosis. What might a new person-centred, ritual-centred language of menopause sound like? A language of tenderness and care, of respect and richness of knowing? How might such language shift our perceptions and experiences? It is worth reminding ourselves, as Lynne Franks does in discussing the wise woman (Chapter 19), that menopause as a health issue is not the only way of characterising the changes that occur as we humans age.

Menopause has come to be understood mainly as a confluence of hormonal changes, commonly categorised into three stages: perimenopause, which can last for a number of years as the hormone balance shifts, stops, starts, stutters; menopause, when periods have ended (often recognised as when there have been no periods for a year); and postmenopause, when, although hormones may have levelled out, changes continue as we age (see the Menopause Literacy section for medical as well as common usage of these terms). There is also hormonal menopause, deliberately induced by blocking oestrogen and sometimes by prescribing other hormones; and surgical menopause, where the womb and sometimes also ovaries are removed. Several chapters in this book relate different experiences of the deliberate withdrawal of female sex hormones. Cat Chong's friend Paige (not their real name) talks about hormonally induced menopause and Lee Hurley voices the often unheard issues of female-to-male transition (Chapter 9).

As Dr Padmini Murthy discusses in her global view of menopause, human rights, and social and anthropological research (Chapter 2), women of different ethnicities and in different countries can experience symptoms in a multitude of ways. These variations can be cultural, so that where older women are more valued, or have greater freedom or power than those of childbearing age, they may experience menopause as a more positive change. However, it is worth noting that greater respect and freedom for older women in a community does not necessarily mean a valuing of older *womanhood*: Dr Eleanor Nwadinobi, president of the Medical Women's International Association (MWIA), highlights, through a personal anecdote, how it can in fact be that women of this age are seen as, or more like, 'men' and this is where the respect comes from (Chapter 14). Patriarchal power structures have not necessarily been dissolved or challenged.

Variances in symptoms may also involve physiological and dietary factors; for example, women in Japan consume large amounts of phytoestrogens and also report fewer hot flushes and night sweats than women in North America. The lack of a specific term for menopause in Japanese is often mentioned and became noted in the West particularly through the writing of anthropologist Margaret Lock, who spent a decade researching the subject. Where there is no specific word in a language for a condition of being, we need to be careful: it could be because it is not experienced, or because it is understood within a different social context; however, it may also be because it is under-recognised or under-valued.

Income level, social position, sexual orientation, cultural background, ethnicity, primary relationships, work, support networks, self-image – all of these will feed into and form our experience of menopause, along with our ability or desire to access medical treatments for problematic symptoms. The differences in access to appropriate healthcare can be shocking: Clare Barstow, for example, exposes the ways in which women in the UK criminal justice system have been appallingly let down (Chapter 10).

We will also be affected by our relationship to fertility and motherhood. Menopause for someone with no children, or who had wanted more children, may bring very different emotions and accommodations than for someone who is a parent comfortable with the size of their family. It can carry a particularly poignant grief for those who have longed for children but been unable to conceive or carry to term. Tessa Sanderson (Chapter 21) speaks movingly and frankly about her journey through IVF, and how, after menopause, she decided to adopt. However, even where the desire for parenthood has not been so close to one's heart, menopause itself can trigger an unexpectedly shocking recognition of this loss. It is also worth remembering that early menopause – or premature ovarian insufficiency (POI), as it is called in the medical terminology – and other gynaecological or hormonal difficulties can afflict much younger people, bringing that loss into years when there can often be an assumption that the ability to become pregnant is a given.

'In Ireland I am hearing from more young women with POI, which supports the growing evidence that it is on the increase,' menopause educator Catherine O'Keeffe told me. She continued:

POI occurs under the age of 40 and can happen as early as your teen-age years. The ovaries stop producing eggs, generally years before they should. The ovaries also stop producing oestrogen and progesterone and so menopause commences. It is further compounded by the fact the ovaries often don't stop fully – they can fluctuate over time. So, as in peri-menopause, a period, ovulation and even pregnancy can occur, but this is at a much younger age, and for pregnancy the statistics are much lower – 5–10% of women with POI may still conceive.

As those with POI can be very young, there are long-term health concerns that need particular focus and attention, for example, heart, bone and brain health. 'The Daisy Network in the UK is a fantastic support for POI and I run the Irish support network for this group,' says Catherine (see page 188). 'I often say to women, if they find natural menopause a challenge then POI and surgical induced menopause come with a harder burden. Who of us would like to be experiencing hot flushes at the age of 15? And this does not touch on the psychological impacts of POI. Much more needs to be done to educate women on POI and ensure we have the right supports in place.'

Each person will also have their own particular blend of hormones, their own individual menstrual cycle, their own perception of themselves and what it means to be a woman (or man) against which to judge whether men-opause brings relief or anguish, new curse or new freedom, or not a great deal of change at all. I myself had probably always been ambivalent about gender. I did not relish the idea of being a woman, and in the years of my childhood and early secondary school, I had not needed to consider myself in that way. As an only child, learning from father as well as mother, feeling their dual support and bearing their twin ambitions, I had received the message that I could go wherever my own capabilities and hard work took me; it was as though I would be excused from sexism. In my voracious reading, I cast myself as the knight, not the princess; I would be Galahad, not Guinevere. Over the years since, I have explored, been troubled by, experimented with, come to love, forgotten about, accepted and wrangled with being a woman, and all that this has entailed in personal life, society and culture in Britain from the late 1970s to 2020. This is the context of my own menopause.

Carol Russell writes eloquently (in Chapter 4) of the rage and grief brought to the surface by her questioning of the memory talents that have been central to her identity as a storyteller, and by societal attitudes: 'At this time in my life, society doesn't expect me to want to achieve the dreams that have been deferred by my womanhood and my African descent, but instead it would prefer me to take a step back and allow the young to have their turn.'

Menopause is not the neat cut-off that the term itself or medical definition suggest. Not just hormones; not only an end of menstruation. It is also, as Sophia Tzeng contemplates (Chapter 5), a shift in our relationship with mortality, with ageing, with our bodies and their rhythms. We also need to question what is collected into the 'bundle' of what we are referring to in our day-to-day use of the word: what is down to menopause and what is about midlife? What is hormonal shift and what is life shift? What aspects of our experience are more about the ongoing progressions of ageing than a single event or condition – especially one that is often characterised as a 'lack': a loss of oestrogen and loss of youth and fertility?

The time of menopause can also be about a transformation of energies – of wanting change, of needing energy to move things that are stuck. A time of risks and of surprise – of being surprised by ourselves. A time of finding and developing a new voice. In my case, poetry suddenly seemed the only way to adequately express what I was feeling, and this has become a new and welcome direction in my life. For Jennifer Nadel (Chapter 1), co-founder of Compassion in Politics, menopause compelled her to speak out about the injustices in the political and social landscape around her.

It can be a time of questioning existing relationships and either revitalising them or embarking on new ones. Our closest ties can be re-forged or newly forged. Sophie Watkins and Stephen Purvis (Chapter 7) discuss with candour and warmth how their own relationship had to evolve and grow to cope with Sophie's surgery and its aftermath, right from the beginning. We may also review our accepted ideas of our sexuality, or decide to live it more authentically. Carren Strock, for example, points out that the majority of the women she interviewed for her book *Married Women Who Love Women* were in their mid-thirties to mid-fifties when their same-sex feelings became apparent – when many were going through perimenopause or reaching menopause (Chapter 8).

For my generation of women in the UK, and other countries where motherhood is being put off until later (I was a month shy of my fortieth birthday when I had my son) and our elders are living longer, menopause also sits between or overlaps the caregiving roles of mother and daughter.

My son was 6 when I began perimenopause at the age of 46; 11 when my periods stopped in 2015. My parents were in their eighties. For me, the meno-'pause' was that tiniest of gaps between nurturing a young child and taking on increasing care and life responsibilities for my own mother and father. I am most definitely part of the so-called sandwich generation. In some ways, I hardly allowed menopause symptoms any attention at the time: there was too much else going on.

It really sank in, talking with Sandra in our Menopause Café conversation (Chapter 20), that I had been hugely stressed, just not noticing it. I was lucky that my partner and son were understanding and supportive, but in a way I had 'put off' dealing with uncomfortable symptoms because there was no space to recognise or think about them properly; no time to stop and do anything about them. Symptoms around vaginal dryness, painful sex, and what I now realise was probably the beginnings of urinary incontinence, and vulval tissues that had become so thin they suffered small tears if I wasn't careful when washing. It was only later, after I had confided in a sympathetic GP when everything became too much, that I felt able to take stock and look at what I myself might be needing. I know I am not alone in this pushing down of my own health needs. It is something that women have traditionally done, and something that is highlighted particularly starkly in Shad Begum's conversations with women in her Pashtun region of Pakistan (Chapter 6).

In both my own lived experience and the experiences of the many people I've spoken to, it is clear that menopause cannot be defined neatly; but part of the issue we face in demystifying the menopause is wrapped up in the lack of an open and honest conversation about it across the spectrum, from policy-makers and medical practitioners to those going through it.

So why do we struggle so much with the M-word?

Talking about female bodies, and acknowledging their humanity – their pains, their discomforts, their amazing imperfections, their wonderful physicality – has been a taboo across many cultures for many hundreds and thousands of years. Female physicality remains a subject that can be difficult to discuss outside an intimate circle, whether of friends or relatives, or of those strangers we quickly connect with through the discovery of shared life events.

In women's medicine, this taboo, and biases around research and drug testing, gender and ethnicity, and believing (or more precisely, not believing) the lived experience of women who present as patients, have led to misinformation and to women going without essential and even life-saving treatments. Gender bias in medicine, and in data collection and analysis more widely, has been laid bare in works such as Caroline Criado Perez's *Invisible Women* and Gabrielle Jackson's *Pain and Prejudice*. Women have been systematically omitted from clinical trials, even of treatments for women, and female animals not used in relevant experiments (although personally I welcome any omission of animals from experimentation). Jackson cites Maya Dusenbery, who wrote how 'a National Institutes of Health-supported pilot study from Rockefeller University [in the US] that looked at how obesity affected breast and uterine cancer didn't enrol a single woman'. During my research I interviewed Mandu Reid, leader of the Women's Equality Party (WEP) and founder of The Cup Effect, which works to empower women and girls across the world by raising awareness about menstrual cups, and she spoke passionately about this issue:

> The genesis of that problem is something really deeply structural and it is this fact of how research isn't done on female subjects and historically hasn't been done on female subjects to the same degree as male subjects. There is this extraordinary example of a libido drug called Addyi [flibanserin] and the safety testing on this female libido drug was carried out on twenty-three male subjects and two female subjects. Now that for me is a 'poster girl' or poster boy example of exactly what's wrong with our medical system.

Reid also referred to the difference in diagnosis rates between men and women as a further example of the challenges women's healthcare faces: 'I was really alarmed when I learned that despite women visiting the GP significantly more frequently than men do, it will take four and a half years or longer for a woman with cancer to be diagnosed and two and a half years longer for a woman with diabetes to be diagnosed.' There are also numerous worrying examples that come up throughout the book, and these differences are not just found between men and women, but also between women, depending on ethnicity and cultural or socioeconomic background. Dr Christine Ekechi calls for more and better research, pointing out the lack of understanding, for example, of why there is a prevalence of fibroids in Black and Asian women (Chapter 18). Dr Wen Shen, in the same chapter, reflects on the incredibly difficult experiences women have been through and continue to suffer with – when better research, education and attitudes towards women's health could make all the difference.

As well as the paucity of medical dialogue and research, the missing conversation around menopause has personal, social and cultural consequences. When locked in our own concerns, without a communal space to share experiences and be validated in them, anxiety and fear can take hold. Finding a companion on the road of menopause, going through something of what we are going through, can bring the 'oh thank God, it's not just me' moment that a number of people I have spoken to for this book have talked about. It's not just about information, it's about being part of a collective rather than out on our own. In her Menopause Café conversation (Chapter 20), Helen Kemp speaks of finding a 'tribe' among those experiencing menopause.

I have also been struck by the number of people who did not learn about menopause, or even much about menstruation, from their mothers or other older female relatives. In my family, menarche – the beginning of periods – was something my parents were open about. We even went for dinner to mark it as an achievement to celebrate (I was slightly mortified, not appreciating the attention in my mid-teens). Both my mother and father were involved in discussions around puberty and relationships: perhaps unusually in suburban 1970s England, given that they were of the generation who reached adulthood in the recently post-Second World War years, before the so-called 'permissive society'. My mother also talked about menopause, and in particular hot flushes, in her later forties, though not other symptoms that I can recall. (Perhaps hot flushes are the most-recognised symptom of menopause because they are simultaneously prevalent and hard to hide in public.) Going back further, her own mother – my grandmother – had struggles with her mental health, which returned in her late forties and fifties and for which she experienced the harrowing treatment of the day, which included ECT (electroconvulsive therapy). Although there were other factors, I now wonder whether part of her psychological distress may have been prompted by the hormonal turbulence of menopause? How many women, over the decades and centuries, might have been misdiagnosed in this way? How many given inappropriate and even damaging treatments that made matters worse, not better? We come back here to the drastic surgical 'treatments' of the nineteenth century – and the fact that women today can still be dismissed as 'hysterical' when they describe pains and symptoms that a doctor does not readily understand.

For some, the intergenerational silence results from specific cultural and religious traditions and taboos, which are touched upon in chapters throughout the book, and perhaps highlighted most powerfully in the voices of women from Pakistan and Afghanistan. In more secular Western societies, the silence can also be related to the construction of shamefulness and diminishment associated with being a woman, and in particular becoming older as a woman – as Caryn Franklin analyses (Chapter 15). But there is a more widespread disconnect, too, which applies to other areas of what used to be traditionally passed-down knowledge. These days, we turn to YouTube for cookery tips and websites for health advice. We have gained computer memory but lost familial memory – a generalisation, as I know from the fact my own pastry-making skills were passed on to me by my mother, but worth noting in relation to women's health and knowing what and who to trust when it comes to caring for our reproductive and bodily selves. Faye Clarke, one of the Australian nurses who has contributed her experience (Chapter 17), also points out the disconnect brought by colonisation for First Nations people there: 'The impact of colonisation has been difficult in that generational conversations have been interfered with and the knowledge of times past has been interrupted. This has a big impact on future generations of women.'

It feels important to reconnect, so that education is not only what we read in leaflets, but what we share face to face, generation to generation – even if, in the socially distanced times in which I am writing this introduction, in the midst of the spring 2020 coronavirus lockdown, that 'face to face' has to be digitally enabled.

If we don't engage with others, we can become sealed in the bubbles of our own particular demographics, either believing on the one hand that everyone else's experience will be similar to our own, or that other people's lives are 'different' in some essential way. This can lead to damaging assumptions and the perpetuation of prejudices and bias, which need to be actively recognised and countered. In her film-making and advocacy, Afghan-born Arzu Qaderi, for example, challenges the media stereotypes of women in her home country to provide a more nuanced understanding, by talking to Afghan women and sharing their real stories (Chapter 16). Throughout the book, we have conversations and perspectives from the UK and US, from Pakistan, Australia, Italy, Nigeria, Afghanistan, Ireland, Canada, Singapore, which are by turns heartfelt, eye-opening, lyrical, shocking, galvanising and speak to the profound impact menopause can have on all areas of life from the personal to the political, from the social to the economic.

Indeed, it is estimated that 14 million working days a year are lost to the UK economy due to women being unable to work because of menopause. But if we go beyond nation and economy, to look at people's actual lives, what do those figures mean in terms of lost household income, job anxiety, halted career progression, workplace bullying, the gender pay gap? To what extent does menopause – like pregnancy and motherhood – shape and limit the choices people make in their work, and affect how they are perceived in that work? Beyond the stereotypical (and also true) image of the menopausal woman having a hot flush in the boardroom, this is something that has a deep effect on those in all kinds of employment, and unemployment. Recognition of the impact of menopause in the workplace, and steps to address this, are thankfully beginning to be taken seriously, certainly in European countries and the US. Catherine O'Keeffe reports on the new initiatives around women's health in the Republic of Ireland, for example (Chapter 13).

A re-education through listening and talking

Learning and understanding is a collaborative process: it is about a making of knowledge with others; it is a relationship. This relationship may be with people we speak to in person, or with what others are writing in our own time; with collective understandings passed down orally, or with the writings of individuals stretching back through the centuries. It is also a knowledge 'written in the body': in our relationship to our selves. Certainly, this is how I have come to view my own knowledge and understanding about menopause.

In the making of this book, I have spoken to and heard from many people, nudging my understanding forward with each encounter. The book itself has also been developed in relationship with my commissioning editor at

Flint, Jo de Vries, with whom I have talked through ideas and directions, all along the way. We have each of us been changed by the process. As Jo wrote to me, in the final stages of putting together the manuscript:

> One of the most profound things for me has been how much it's made me think about how I've passively accepted so many things about my own menstrual and gynaecological health as being a 'woman's lot'. I now realise how often I've ignored or felt ashamed of so much of that part of being a woman; how little I've educated myself about things that could have been addressed or I could have got help with. Working on this book has really changed my perspective on that and I hope will mean that I can enter the menopause feeling more empowered to ask the right questions and find out information rather than being fobbed off or being too 'frightened' or ashamed to complain.

The need for education and empowerment is a theme that runs through the contributions to this book. As I gathered information myself, I decided I wanted to know more about HRT, since hormone therapies ('replacing' oestrogen and sometimes progesterone) are often the main treatment route offered by GPs and other health professionals. As Dr Shen points out, however, a number of potential symptoms listed for menopause (see page 293) are due to more complex interactions, including lifestyle factors and the ageing process. I also wanted to know why HRT remains far less prescribed, certainly in the UK, in the early twenty-first century than in the 1990s. I had known that I did not want to take so-called systemic HRT (for the whole system, in tablet, gel, patch, or implant form), but I did research and opt for oestrogen pessaries to alleviate the vaginal dryness and skin thinning. I talked to Dr Caroline Marfleet, a consultant in reproductive and sexual health who has specialised in women's health for more than forty years, to discuss this further. Issues around HRT, which was first introduced in 1965, arose with the publication in 2002 of initial findings from the Women's Health Initiative, a clinical trial in the US, and results from the Million Women Study in the UK that came out in 2003. These studies taken together suggested links between types of HRT and increased risk of coronary events, stroke, thrombosis and cancers, in particular breast cancer, although later analysis has questioned some of the risk levels given in initial published findings.

The NHS, said Dr Marfleet, does not have a specific policy to avoid prescribing HRT, but 'some [GP] practices decided against HRT and took a "no risk" approach rather than finding out more'. In part, this was a financial as well as a health decision: they did not want to be called to account in our current 'blame society'. Dr Marfleet pointed out that recent studies show HRT can have preventative and protective aspects for quality of life and moods, osteoporosis, vulvovaginal and urinary issues, and heart disease (if started within ten years of menopause). 'Not all HRT is the same; the types of oestrogens and progestogens used in HRT are now known to have different effects and outcomes on the female system,' she explained. 'There are also different effects depending on the method of delivery as evidence has shown a small increased risk of blood clots with oral HRT, which is generally not seen with transdermal HRT (gels and patches) as these do not pass through the liver.'

HRT is one, hotly debated, way in which menopause has become medicalised in the modern age, and in the past few years there have been more radical developments that may change our definition of it altogether. While the Medical Women's International Association (MWIA) and other organisations define menopause as a natural part of ageing, scientists in Greece have apparently been able to 'reverse' it by 'rejuvenating' the ovaries of menopausal women using a blood plasma treatment. At the same time, many women are continuing with long-term HRT. So, one question is whether we now live in postmenopausal, or even non-menopausal times? Some people advocate an acceptance of menopause as an important stage of life: one that should be ritualised and recognised, and that can bring spiritual maturity and wisdom. For others, HRT has been a lifeline through changes that have undermined their physical and mental health, and relationships. Any questioning of the medicalisation of menopause (and the profits of the pharmaceuticals industry, for example) needs at the same time to prioritise and think through what is important for women's health and well-being.

What of the future? Initiatives that put this reclaiming of women's health at the foreground are beginning to spring up. Dr Shen has set up a new Women's Wellness and Healthy Aging Program at Johns Hopkins in Baltimore, bringing together specialists from the many different areas of health that can be impacted. Mandu Reid, as leader of the Women's Equality Party (WEP), is excitingly proposing a Women's Health Institute in London:

What we're fighting for in London is an acknowledgement of all the ways in which women are disbelieved, misdiagnosed and let down by the health system. And it's the whole cycle – it starts at research, it moves on to diagnosis and it moves on to treatment. In a way women are second-class citizens when it comes to health outcomes that they're on the receiving end of.

We spoke about the need, identified by many contributors to this book, for better training for primary care doctors. 'When GPs are being trained, as part of their core training there need to be modules that are compulsory for them to undertake that are designed and informed not only by those who have medical qualifications but also women who have been through menopause and, crucially, have had to navigate the health system blind spots around how menopause is treated,' said Reid.

She and the WEP are keen to ensure there is a focus not only on the inequalities *for* women, but *between* women. Asked about the differences in health outcomes for BAME women and women in low-income groups, Reid spoke, like Dr Ekechi, about the importance of research. This needs to be high-quality research that will:

Examine and drill down to understand what the source or sources of these inequalities are. We know that in this country Black women are five times more likely to die in childbirth than their white counterparts and I find it devastating to know that that's the case, although I am pleased that someone has studied that. But what's missing are further lines of enquiry and proper research to understand why ... More money needs to be invested in women's health research full stop, but a portion of that cash needs to be ring-fenced as a deliberate, purposeful thing to examine the differences between groups.

This will mean convincing senior medical and clinical practitioners. 'Unfortunately, money talks,' admits Reid. 'But if you look at healthy quality of life, women's healthy quality of life is shorter than men's, even though women live longer in total. Now, if women have a better healthy quality of life that would be better for our families, for our communities and for the economy. So, if somebody needs a business case for this research, then this is it.'

Reid's mother is originally from Malawi, and she herself, with The Cup Effect, works with girls and women in lower-income countries. One of the things that Reid has been passionate about with The Cup Effect is engendering better 'menstrual literacy'. She reflects that:

Actually a 13-year-old girl in Sheffield has a lot more in common with a girl growing up in a rural part of Malawi, when it comes to her attitudes and experiences of menstruation, than I would have thought. So, the shame, the stigma, the embarrassment is really shared by the people in both of those communities. The big difference is really the ready access to menstrual products.

And she feels that this also applies to the menopause:

I think this whole thing of informed choice applies as much to menopause as it does to menstruation. We need menopause literacy too ... It was certainly absent from my education. I'm 39 now and I'm training myself to be vigilant as I know I could be heading for the perimenopausal part of my life, but I didn't even learn the word perimenopause until 2 years ago. Why didn't I learn that when I was a youngster? ... It's really important whether you're talking about puberty or the later periods of your life where your body is changing, so your life is changing.

On the one hand, menopause may be seen as a universalising experience – something all those with female anatomy or hormone cycles will go through, in one form or another – but that doesn't mean putting forward a model of menopause that privileges particular experiences and understandings. From the outset, the aim of this collection has been to bring together voices from different walks of life and cultural backgrounds, to begin unravelling and listening to the complex, difficult, worrying, poignant, creative variety of lived experiences.

As with the menstrual movement before it, the debate and the mood around menopause are changing. In the past few years, there has been a shift – something that Rachel Weiss reflects on (Chapter 20), when talking about setting up the groundbreaking and now international Menopause

Café movement. There is a growing body of people and websites providing support, campaigning, making menopause matter to the wider population – people like Diane Danzebrink, founder of the #MakeMenopauseMatter campaign in the UK (Chapter 3), Catherine O'Keeffe, who extended this campaign to Ireland, and Aisling Grimley, who set up the My Second Spring website from her home in the Republic of Ireland (Chapter 13).

The aim of this book is to open up the exchange of conversations about menopause, so that they can take place not only in local gatherings, whether in person or online, but internationally, by reaching out to people across the globe. It is not a 'how to' manual or advice book – although you may find the stories of those here strike a chord in mapping your own menopause and deciding what might be helpful or necessary for you. It is based on an understanding of menopause as unique for every person; there are commonalities that reach across continents, and at the same time stark differences within families – between mother and daughter, sister and sister. This book is also based on a belief that all of us, whatever our gender or assigned sex, could benefit from understanding more about that variety of experience. Menopause as not just a 'women's problem', but something social, cultural, familial and a fact of life that affects almost everyone in some way: as sister, brother, friend, partner, child, or as someone going through it.

This book is only a beginning, however, and there is only so much it has been able to cover in these pages: there need to be more and wider conversations; more women, men and non-binary people of different backgrounds and experiences brought to the table, having their contributions valued and listened to. There needs to be a range of culturally appropriate safe spaces in which we feel able express and share, and discover what will be helpful in our own particular context. We also need places and networks to debate and grow what can and should be done on a broader societal and global level.

In exploring the physical and very human geography of menopause, putting this book together, talking to and virtually 'meeting' with people around the globe, I have learned so much, both about other people's experiences of menopause, health and ill health, their lives and hopes, and also about my own understanding of menopause. I hope that, as readers, it touches and empowers you too.

This book is dedicated to my mother, June Marjorie Harris (June 1931–April 2019), and to her mother, and her mother, and her mother ... and to all of our future generations.

Caroline Harris
May 2020

Caroline Harris is an author, educator, publisher and poet. With more than twenty-five years' experience in journalism and publishing, she began her career at feminist magazine *Spare Rib* and spent seven years with *The Observer*. More recently, she co-founded book creation business Harris + Wilson and has lectured in publishing, including as Course Leader for the BA Publishing at Bath Spa University. She is the author of *Ms Harris's Book of Green Household Management* (John Murray) and young adult novel *Consequences: Holding the Front Page* (Hodder Children's). Her debut poetry pamphlet, *SCRUB Management Handbook No.1 Mere*, is published by Singing Apple Press. She currently lives in Bath with her partner and son, and is studying for a PhD in poetic practice at Royal Holloway, University of London. Her interests range from yoga to deer, cycling to ecological philosophy, women's lives to the life of words.

1

It's Time to Make 'Normal' Visible

Compassion in Politics founder and bestselling author of *WE: A Manifesto for Women Everywhere*, Jennifer Nadel explores how the menopause turned her life upside down and set her out on a new path.

I've just finished writing my first novel. It's the spring of 2010 and I've been invited to read from it at a conference hosted by one of my writing heroes – an attractive, distinguished and celebrated male novelist. The conference's theme is sex. So, I begin to read the scene where my 15-year-old female narrator loses her virginity. I'm comfortable with the material. I'm confident reading in public. But within seconds of standing up, I feel myself flush deep red and beads of sweat begin to form on my forehead. By the end of the reading I have sweat running down my face. I must look as if I've just finished running a marathon. Those around me – including my literary heart throb – comfort me, assuming it has been a traumatic ordeal to read so explicitly about sex in public. They were wrong. It was, I now know, my first hot flush.

I was unprepared. Like the girl in the shower at the start of *Carrie*, who becomes hysterical when she discovers she is bleeding because she doesn't know about periods, I knew nothing about this biological and inevitable process. A process whereby my periods would dry up and I would begin an intense and largely uncontrollable biological, intellectual and spiritual journey.

In my forties, the menopause wasn't something any of my normally liberal friends had discussed. My initial shock and embarrassment soon gave way to fascination. I was intrigued that my body could suddenly and unexpectedly generate so much heat. I had a new superpower. I could go from cold to boiling in no time at all. My body had become an out-of-control radiator that would suddenly perform its turbo-charged stunt without warning. At night, I'd wake to find my sheets sodden. Pools of sweat would collect on my chest between my breasts. My hair would be drenched.

But the hot flushes were the least of it.

To accompany them came all manner of hormonal shifts, not dissimilar to a second puberty. Mood swings. Uncontrollable rage. A loss of control. I found myself furious over the smallest thing, sometimes aware that I was overreacting, sometimes not, but never able to stop myself once I'd started. I couldn't explain how my personality had changed so dramatically. For my first forty-eight years on this planet I'd been dismissive about all things domestic. And now, here I was raging about the cutlery. My children started to walk on eggshells, and I began to wonder if I'd had an unrecognised head injury or perhaps a brain tumour. At the same time, I noticed a diminishing of maternal feelings: a hardening in the heart area. For the first time, I became able to loosen my vampiric grip on my offspring. I went from smother-mother to laissez-faire in lightning speed: 'They'll work it out' replaced 'How am I going to make this better for them?'

At the same time came a desire to be free – to upend my life and finally give it a full and true expression. I was well aware of the privileges in my life, as a middle-class, cis, professionally educated white woman, but I was overcome by a deep dissatisfaction with the state of things in the world and haunted by a feeling that whatever I had done was not enough. I felt that I was surrounded by phoneys – a throwback to my adolescent rage against the hypocrisy of all things. I felt an urgent need to remedy the situation, accompanied by a gnawing dread that change was now impossible: it was too late.

There was also a crippling anxiety, out of all proportion to the task at hand. I found myself at an airport one day about to leave for a holiday with close girlfriends but unable to get on the plane, sobbing and seized by an unexplainable terror. A haziness took hold of my brain. I used to think I was reasonably intelligent, but now I lost the car on a regular basis and forgot close friends' names. I could no longer be sure that if I started to express an opinion my brain would be able to marshal the facts I knew were there to back it up. My kids booked me in for dementia testing; luckily I didn't qualify but it was close.

I had been privileged with a good education, but still I knew nothing. It took me the first few years to piece together the many disparate ways in which the menopause was affecting me.

Physically there were more seemingly unrelated symptoms. Like the thinning of my hair, which would fall out by the handful. I thought I was going bald and not just on my head – eyebrows, lashes and elsewhere as well. Sunburn down the parting became a thing and, like a middle-aged man, I had to start wearing hats in the sun. Simultaneously, hairs grew unbidden in all sorts of random and unwelcome places. Those occasional mole hairs doubled in size. They could now appear unpredictably almost anywhere, obliging me to make a coma-pact with my best friend – a recip-rocal agreement to tweeze out the worst offenders if either of us should end up paralysed. The snowy down of an early adolescent boy appeared on my cheek and chin. Nostril hair, it turned out, was not just for hirsute men. My skin lost its elasticity; my stomach became distended, my boobs emptied. My periods stopped and then returned heavier than ever. A last desperate throw of the dice by a cycle that knew it was on the way out. Stress inconti-nence was now not just for trampolines but for any energetic activity when my bladder hadn't been fully emptied. Scaly, old-person skin emerged on my legs. Everything began to dry out.

Then, when the penny finally dropped, came the panic over HRT. Would it cause cancer? Would it give me a stroke?

I resisted the very idea of it to start with. This was a natural process, I argued; surely I should feel and learn whatever lesson was buried in it? But, like childbirth, not all of us can rely on our breath. Some of us need medical intervention and extra help. As the symptoms ramped up and my unexplained mood swings took their toll on an already wobbling marriage, I succumbed to the idea that I might not be able to manage this myself.

By this point, those friends who could afford to were spending small fortunes on alternative therapies. I myself visited a string of passionately rec-ommended 'experts' who prescribed a cocktail of creams that would be mixed specially for me in another country. One such 'expert' suggests that rubbing these creams into my labia will bring me heightened sexual pleasure in a way that makes me feel this is more about his sexual gratification than mine.

When I've put myself into my overdraft, I realise that not only can I not be sure that any of these so-called treatments have actually made a difference, but that I'm also starting to sink into a depression. I end up in my GP's surgery. She wins me over when she tells me that it isn't just my skin that is drying up but also my organs. Hormones can actually keep me younger internally. She persuades me that a good old NHS prescription of conventional hormones is in fact much safer, as it's been tested in ways that bioidentical hormones have not. I surrender, take the gel and pills she prescribes and start to feel human again.

Many of my close friends still swear by their alternative bioidentical remedies, even though the British Menopause Society has clearly withheld its approval for them, emphasising on its website that they are not evidence-based or regulated. Each of us must choose the path which works best for us, but I give thanks every day for the simplicity and effectiveness of my NHS regime, which my wonderful GP tells me that, all things being equal, I'll be able to continue with into my seventies.

Now I find myself a modern-day Ancient Mariner, trapping any woman I encounter who is perimenopausal, to disgorge my new-found knowledge. To warn them of what is to come. So that they, unlike me, will arrive on menopausal shores prepared and will know to head straight to their doctor.

But the physiological and hormonal aspects are just one part of the story.

Layered on top of our individual journey through 'the change', as it was ominously referred to by my mother's generation, are mythical narratives that do little to ease our passage. Take the stereotypes that society projects onto women who are beyond childrearing age. We become crones, hags, spinsters. As women, most of us have battled throughout our adult lives (no matter how strong our feminism) with the cultural imperatives to look a certain way. Billions of dollars are spent every year to convince us as women (and increasingly men too) that we are not OK as we are. That we need to be thinner, look younger, act sexier. We need to buy clothes, bags, miracle creams. We need to groom and corral ourselves into some preset notion of desirability if we want to gain acceptance.

From the moment we can toddle, society grooms us to self-objectify: from Cinderella and Sleeping Beauty to *Friends* and *Love Island*. As humans we are biologically programmed to fit into our tribe. In early times exclusion or being on the edge of the herd spelt death. And, socially and emotionally, it can still feel like that. So, it's hardly surprising that from puberty (and increasingly before) so many of us try to contort and twist ourselves to fit the norms with which society imprisons us.

We may think we're more liberated now, but look at how many of us sexualise ourselves in ways that feminists a generation ago would never have countenanced. The women's libbers who marched and fought for the right for us all not to be objectified and defined by our 'femaleness' have given way to a generation who find themselves obliged to spend more time on personal grooming than ever before. Take the incredible growth of nail bars, brow bars, blow-dry bars – all catering to a demand to look as perfect as the airbrushed icons of our day.

Somewhere along the way, we've mistaken our ability to self-objectify as a choice and say it brings us freedom and power. We take up pole- and lap-dancing. We say we feel powerful and in control of our sexuality, when all too often, really we are finishing the patriarchy's work for them. Teetering on heels that throw our backs out and destroy our feet, those of us who can afford to (and many who can't) pay millions for new breasts, fuller lips and tauter skin. We inject poison into our faces. One of the fastest-growing areas of demand in plastic surgery is for labiaplasty, a direct result of porn's influence. Even our labia and vaginas need to fit the male gaze.

And then what happens? Smack, bang: we hit a certain age (that like the horizon seemed always to be vanishing but then suddenly isn't) and the whole house of cards upon which we've consciously (or unconsciously) constructed our femaleness comes tumbling down. Just as societal and cultural norms had us believe that our earlier female worth was inextricably bound up with our sexual desirability, now they have us believing that once our fertile years are gone we will inevitably be cast aside – unwanted, dried-up husks. Alongside that myth comes another, that once menopausal we become invisible to men and are inevitably passed over in favour of younger, more succulent flesh. Evidence abounds of the ways in which at work, too, many of us are edged out and replaced by younger models. The fate of some of those who have taken up the fight against ageism in the workplace is hardly encouraging. Take former BBC *Countryfile* presenter Miriam O'Reilly, who won her age discrimination court case against the BBC but was then not offered any work commensurate with her experience and status.

It is a brutal barrier to hit. And it hits many of us hard. It did me. It strips away what we thought was our identity. And if we are not to accept the rather uninviting storylines that society offers us, we have to be willing to take the path less travelled and rebuild ourselves from the inside out. The challenge is not just about shaking off the patriarchal stories we have internalised and then often made real. If we listen to its invitation, the menopause offers us an opportunity to discover who we are, naked of biological drivers and shorn of the capacity to pretend towards youth. With this change comes the chance to discover who we are beneath the roles and identities we have adopted.

Accompanying that invitation, a related siren sounds – a klaxon that calls us to consider our own mortality. It summons to the surface a host of existential conundrums. Questions that most of us have become adept at suppressing or dodging and may have made their last appearance during the metaphysical angst of our late adolescence, in my case in the early 1980s when my heroes were Sartre, Beckett and Camus. What are we here for? Is there any meaning to anything that we do? What abides? What's the point? The questions remind us that the longest stretch of our life is now behind us. That just as our puberty signalled the beginning of our fertile years, the menopause has called time on them. We are being shunted forward on the conveyor belt of life as our biological function falls away. The challenge is not to allow ourselves to fall with it.

And that, ironically, is where some of the symptoms of the menopause become its solutions. That is where our irritability and intolerance can be called into service. Where those of us who experience a falling away of our more maternal instincts can harness that to drive change. We are given the chance to no longer have to accept the definitions we've been given. To cast aside labels and stereotypes that limit and diminish us. To start to say no, instead of yes. To start to say 'Not for me', rather than 'How lovely, thank you'.

We stand at a crossroads. We can capitulate to the myths that menopause carries and enter death's antechamber. Or we can declare ourselves free at last and begin to prioritise what really matters to us in the time that is available. With no myths left that will serve and carry us forward in a positive direction we have to create our own. We are called to reject narratives founded on drying up, invisibility and witchcraft. This is the moment when we can start to write and create our own myths, role models and archetypes.

The hormonal rollercoaster and the existential angst that the menopause ushers in become the crucible where we get to choose our new identity. It's a time when we can own our sexuality, free at last from the fear of an unwanted conception. If we want, sex can become just sex. It is no longer about procreation. With inhibitions lessened and the wisdom of an elder, we can fully step into our sexuality in ways we may not yet have been able to. Or, we can stop wanting sex. Loss of libido (along with vaginal dryness and repeated urinary tract infections) is a common hormonal side-effect. I have a number of friends, married and not, who have happily declared themselves celibate and extol the virtues of the freedom that it brings. Just as with adolescence, the hormonal shifts of the menopause can embolden us to take risks and make changes. Other friends have come out, had wild affairs, declared themselves done with motherhood. The story of midlife menopausal crisis has been largely focused on men. But we women have our stories too and, tellingly, more women leave their marriages or long-term relationships than men during this period.

It is now that many of us find our voice and start to say what was previously unsayable. To outgrow the constraints of our fraught childhoods and the complications of our middle years to blossom finally as our true selves. For my own part, I have felt fear fall away. I've found myself able to speak out and champion causes without inhibition where previously self-consciousness held me back. Talking and writing about the menopause, for example, would have had my younger self cringing. Since that literary conference when I stood humiliated and dripping in the sweat of my first hot flush, I've found myself running for parliament and revealing my struggle with depression to millions on TV. I've also overcome many of the constraints of my childhood. I came from a 'good girls don't talk' home where the rule was not to speak and never to reveal anything personal. The menopause well and truly smashed that rule. It isn't that I've belatedly located a pocket of bravery, it's simply that I don't care anymore. I don't care what you think of me. But there are lots of things I do really care about and they have risen to the top – the truth, injustice, refugees, climate change and fighting to end avoidable suffering. That insecurity which dogged my fertile years has withered on the vine. And it feels amazing.

It is not just marriages that get upended during this period, it can be friendships as well. I've watched and experienced splits with long-term female friends. Quirks and traits that have long been seen as sweet or endearing suddenly become intolerable. Simultaneously, old friends reappear from nowhere. Just at the moment that a close friend stops talking to me a best friend from decades ago miraculously makes contact. Increasingly, I find myself slipping back into stride with friends I was last close to in my twenties as if the thirty intervening years had never happened. It increasingly feels as if we are in some giant game of musical chairs with the music slowing down and all of us trying to position ourselves where we want to be when the music stops.

For many of us there is also a growing intolerance for bad behaviour or unkindness. In my case, that intolerance resulted in the setting up of Compassion in Politics, a not-for-profit which fights for the rights of the most vulnerable. For me, as for many others, the sight of refugees dying at sea, the rise in homelessness and food banks in a wealthy, civilised nation is an abomination. There are some incredibly commonsense fixes which could dramatically reduce avoidable suffering, like, for example, ensuring that laws can't be passed if they make those in the most vulnerable circumstances worse off. Compassion is innate to all humans and yet somehow our politicians have allowed it to be eclipsed by greed and the pursuit of infinite growth. Compassion in Politics aims to anchor politics to the values of kindness and empathy that most of us live by.

Increasingly, the menopause enables us to stop bending our shape to fit the other's projections; instead we own our truth. It takes practice. Like learning to walk, it requires stumbles and falls. We may overextend ourselves. My first bout of menopausal activism, in the run-up to the climate change talks in 2009, left me burnt out. We may see fights where there are none. But we are each other's midwives. We cheer each other on to take whichever path our soul dictates.

Menopause is both a crisis and an opportunity. But for too long it has remained hidden in the shadows, a subject of shame or ignorance. It is time that we as women begin to own it publicly for the rite of passage that it is. It is time to cast away the misconceptions, the shame and the stigma. And to celebrate the potential the menopause gives us to stand in the full glory of our power.

The #MeToo movement has shown how longstanding attitudes and behaviours can begin to shift. It is time for us to start campaigning for attitudes around the menopause to shift too. In *WE: A Manifesto for Women Everywhere*, the bestselling book I co-wrote with Gillian Anderson, we call for all women who have the privilege of being able to speak out to use it. It's time to start telling it as it is. To talk about the reality of what it is to be female. Not to pretend that we are only the groomed and scented versions of ourselves that we project. No longer to remain silent for fear of making ourselves unacceptable or unloveable. We need to make the normal visible, otherwise we will forever remain trapped in stereotypes that don't serve us. We need to ensure that proper information about the options is available for anyone struggling with the menopause's hormonal impact, and that all GPs are properly trained to understand just how debilitating the symptoms can be. But at the same time, let's be careful not just to medicalise it and leave it as a 'woman's problem' that needs solving. Let's use it also as an opportunity to cast aside the stigmatising and unhelpful tropes that for too long have constrained us and to celebrate all that we are: fully embodied, real and wonderful women.

Jennifer Nadel is an author, poet, activist, award-winning journalist and co-founder of Compassion in Politics (compassioninpolitics.com), which works to put compassion at the centre of public policy. As a journalist she reported for the BBC, Channel 4 and ITV from around the world. Her report on the use of rape as a weapon of war in Bosnia was used by war crimes investigators and her book on domestic violence is credited with helping to shift the law and was made into a BBC film and a Channel 4 documentary. Her most recent book, the Sunday Times bestseller *WE: A Manifesto for Women Everywhere*, was co-authored with Gillian Anderson and is a guide for those seeking spiritual growth and to make a difference in the world. She has run for the UK parliament twice, speaks internationally and lives in London with her three sons.

2

Menopause:
A Human Rights Issue

Dr Padmini Murthy, a trained obstetrician and gynaecologist, is Professor and Global Health Director at the New York Medical College School of Health Sciences and Practice. She is Global Health Lead of the American Medical Women's Association and First Vice President of the Global NGO Executive Committee associated with the Department of Global Communications to the United Nations. She explores how her work with women across the globe has shown her how important menopause is as a human rights issue.

> Gender is a 'lens' through which to consider the appropriateness of various policy options and how they will affect the well-being of both women and men ...
>
> *Active Ageing: A Policy Framework*, World Health Organization (2002)

Menopause is one of the most important reproductive health issues for women, but is not discussed openly due to many social and cultural factors. A natural occurrence associated with the ageing process for women, menopause is characterised by the cessation of periods and can impact women's reproductive and sexual health. Most women experience menopause between the ages of 45 and 54, with the average age of menopause being 51. As longevity globally increases, women are living longer after reaching menopause, but often do not have the support and medical services they need. In addition to this lack of support networks, in many societies, women are devalued at the onset of menopause, because of its impact on their fertility and childbearing. As a result of rising life expectancy, by the year 2030 the World Bank estimates that the global population of menopausal women will be around 1.2 billion.

Many factors can influence the health of women during their life cycle and impact the way they deal with this important menopause milestone. A review of research findings published in the *International Journal of Women's Medicine* at the end of 2019 noted that these can include family support, educational level, employment, economic status, marital status, the number of pregnancies she has had and her childbirthing experiences.

A global overview of culture and menopause

It is ironic that in 2020, as the world is celebrating the seventy-fifth anniversary of the United Nations and the twenty-fifth year since the Beijing Declaration from the Fourth World Conference on Women 'determined to advance the goals of equality, development and peace for all women everywhere in the interest of all humanity', women continue to suffer in silence, in spite of shouldering so much of the socioeconomic responsibility in the communities and societies they live in.

As a healthcare professional – a physician and public health professional – working in the area of women's health issues for the past thirty years, I have myself come across taboos and discrimination against menopausal women. Unfortunately, the challenges associated with 'climacteric', as menopause is referred to, have not been addressed and have not been included in policies for women, while social norms have not taken into account the tremendous emotional, physical and psychological issues women face during this phase of their lives. Whenever I have the opportunity, I include the topic of menopause in conversations with both women and men, even at social gatherings. In the past two years, I have noticed the subtle change in attitude, as people – especially men – who are not shocked or horrified, engage in discussions on menopause.

In recent years, menopause has been included on the agenda of the World Health Organization, related to women's health and well-being. The theme of the World Health Day organised by the World Health Organization in 2012 was 'Good Health Adds Life to Years' and a report published by the Department of Reproductive Health and Research on sexual health in older women clearly states that:

> Regardless of their marital status, women of all ages have a right to sexual health, defined by the World Health Organization (WHO) as a state of physical, mental and social well-being in the sphere of sexuality. Intrinsic to the right to sexual health are a positive and respectful approach to sexuality and sexual relationships, as well as the possibility of having sexual experiences that are pleasurable and safe, free from coercion, discrimination, violence and disease.

The attitudes towards and treatment of women who are menopausal are influenced by the traditions, culture and prevailing beliefs in the communities they live and work in. For example, in many Western countries, medical terms such as 'ovarian failure' can be used in some instances to describe the cause of infertility associated with premature menopause. This illustrates the medicalisation of menopause, instead of viewing it as a natural phenomenon occurring at any age. Furthermore, in these cultures importance is often placed more on looking youthful and attractive than on loss of fertility. Unfortunately, women in industrialised countries such as the US and UK have silently suffered the onset of menopause and the postmenopausal period in their lives. Research undertaken in the UK and published by the British Menopause Society in October 2017 found that 45 per cent of women surveyed indicated that their menopausal symptoms had a negative impact on their work. Of those who needed to take a day off work, 47 per cent said they would not specify the exact reason to their employer. From my experience as a health professional, talking to women, this is especially the case with male bosses, due to lack of understanding and the stigma associated with the issue.

The societal attitudes and environment in which a woman lives also play an important role in her own understanding and experience when dealing with menopause. According to a 2015 Reuters article, researchers found in a multicultural study of older women and men living in North America and Europe that the symptoms of menopause, both physical and mental, reported by women can be attributed to language differences, prevailing attitudes and culturally influenced gender roles, as well as the prevailing social and economic conditions. Interestingly, there was considerable variation between countries with similar environments and cultures. For example, women surveyed in Denmark, Sweden and Norway had a more positive view of menopause in comparison to women from the US, the UK, Canada and France.

Studies have also investigated differing perceptions in other regions of the world. For example, a 2015 study in *The Iranian Journal of Obstetrics, Gynecology and Infertility* reported how Mayan women are respected as elders when they enter menopause. In this culture, ageing raises the status of a woman and she is exempt from her routine chores, which are taken over by younger women. In some cultures, such as the Mayan, women consider attaining menopause as a freedom and and it is not medicalised as it is in some others. Another study cited in *Menopause in Cultural Context* related how Chinese women are of the opinion that when they attain menopause, they are reborn, as they can save their energy, which they believe was lost during childbirth. It is interesting to note that Chinese women seldom use drugs or hormonal supplements to reduce menopausal symptoms. Chinese women I have spoken to outside the US are also influenced by their cultural beliefs with regard to menopause and have expressed feelings of relief once they attain this stage, since they feel re-energised and can devote themselves to other pursuits, including meditation and pursuing volunteerism and spiritual activities.

Research also shows that religion or a strong set of spiritual beliefs or faith can have a beneficial impact on menopause. Studies have examined the positive impact of prayer and religion on people's attitudes and acceptance of life, health challenges and menopause in some cultures. To illustrate this further, according to a 2014 article in *Advances in Nursing and Midwifery*, Iranian women consider menopause as a natural phenomenon which is predetermined in a woman's life cycle by God. They may consider it as a blessing, as they can pray uninterrupted without being considered unclean, due to the cessation of their menstrual period, and can have a sexual relationship without fear of any accidental pregnancy.

However, globally (especially in many conservative societies), discussion about sexual behaviour among menopausal women is still frequently a taboo and prevailing societal norms can be a barrier to women seeking advice and counselling for sexual dysfunction and symptoms of dyspareunia (pain during sex) and vaginal dryness. Often women are not aware that the sexual problems which can manifest during menopause can be addressed by looking to medical services instead of suffering in silence. In the UK, the British Menopause Society study found that 51 per cent of women surveyed said the onset of menopause affected their sex life, while 28 per cent of partners of menopausal women reported that they often had arguments, as they did not understand the challenges these women faced.

Lifestyle, education and menopause

India is one of the world's most populated countries and has undergone rapid changes in many fields in the past thirty years. There are around 65 million women in India over the age of 45, and the average age of menopause is 46 years. That being said, as with elsewhere in the world, there are women in the age range of 30–35 who can start experiencing the symptoms of menopause prematurely. According to estimates, by 2050, 20 per cent of the Indian population will be over 60 years of age.

Most of the public health systems relating to women in India are stretched thin, as they have been set up to address the issues and challenges related to childbirth, menstrual disorders and puberty, along with infectious and chronic diseases, rather than menopause. Private clinics and hospitals are expensive, and a majority of the population cannot afford these services. But whether private or public, the healthcare infrastructure is not designed to address the specific health challenges of older women, especially menopause, and this leads to their neglect. A lack of family and society support is coupled with a lack of awareness, low literacy levels, poverty, gender bias and discrimination. These factors, along with the difficulties of accessing healthcare facilities, are barriers to women accepting menopause as an integral part of their life cycle. Indeed, especially in rural areas, most women are not well informed about menopause and many are of the opinion that it is an unavoidable disease.

Evidence-based studies, including research from Iran published in *The Iranian Journal of Obstetrics, Gynecology and Infertility* and from South Korea revealed in *The Journal of Korean Medical Science*, have highlighted the inverse relationship between awareness of menopause and the severity of menopausal symptoms. To illustrate this further: studies in these two countries found that women with lower education levels were at a greater risk of experiencing severe symptoms in comparison to women who had higher levels of education and awareness. One reason for this is that women with more education are more likely to have strategies to address the onset of menopause and to seek support (medical or social) as the need arises. It is also worth noting that the average age for the onset of menopause was found to be higher in more educated women.

However, the global picture can be contradictory. For example, 2005 data from Taiwan found that women with higher levels of education indicated they had more challenges with the onset of menopause than women with less education. Whereas other studies have found that women from both the East and the West who had higher education levels had a less stressful experience and more positive attitude towards menopausal changes (including peri- and postmenopause). Meanwhile, the study of women in South Korea already mentioned, published in 2010, found that among those living in urban areas, women with a higher education level reported milder symptoms of menopause.

Societal support and the workplace

A study published in 1994 in *Maturitas* surveyed a cohort of more than 1,500 Australian women; the results indicated that women in a stable relationship were better able to deal with menopause symptoms, compared to women who were separated, widowed or single. This reiterates the positive influence of a good support system in helping women cope with the onset and duration of menopause. Employment status also significantly affected the experience of menopause symptoms. There is a range of explanations for this finding, which has come across in a number of studies around the world. Being employed may act as a stress buffer for some women who are approaching menopause. Employed women also seem to have more opportunities, financial independence and access to services, including joining support groups outside the home, and thus report milder menopause symptoms. The finding also suggests a positive correlation between the employment status of menopausal women and their psychological well-being, and that being employed is helpful in dealing with this stage of their lives positively.

However, this does not mean to say there aren't issues within the workplace. Menopause brings a tremendous economic burden of millions of pounds every year because employers don't understand it, according to a 2017 government report in the UK. The report, from the Government Equalities Office, indicated that one in ten women in their early fifties suffer 'severe symptoms' as a result of menopause, which affect their work. A conservative estimate highlighted that the absence from work of these 174,200 women aged between 50 and 54 due to menopause symptoms affected the economy by at least £7.3 million in 'absence-related costs'. This figure did not include costs attributed to late arrival of employees due to medical appointments during working hours or reduction in the number of working hours as a result of menopause. The report, entitled 'Menopause transition: effects on women's economic participation', made a strong recommendation that managers and other senior administrative staff in organisations needed to understand menopause and be made aware of the need for addressing menopause-related issues in the workplace.

Unlike institutional guidelines for pregnant workers or for maternity leave, there is seldom a discussion and specific policy provided for addressing menopause in the workplace globally. The UK report further released some troubling evidence of women being harassed, made fun of and subjected to criticism by superiors and colleagues in the workplace as a result of their menopausal symptoms. The terms used to describe older women included being 'hysterical', 'histrionic' or 'menopausal-ish'. The groundbreaking report stressed the need for strong social responsibility and for increased organisational attention to the menopausal transition, to enable middle-aged women to have access to a high quality of working life, similar to that available to colleagues. It made an important observation that 'gendered ageism seems to be the cause of many of the problems which working women experience during transition. This requires changes in prevailing values, beliefs and norms in organisations.'

Reports and findings from the US published in a 2019 Quartz article also demonstrate how menopause and perimenopause can have an impact on women's working lives. According to 2017 data from the US National Institute on Ageing, perimenopause typically begins between 45 and 55, and can last between seven and fourteen years. In 2018, there were around

15.5 million women employed in the US in the 44–55 age group, according to the US Bureau of Labor, and 33.2 million women of 45 and over. These figures illustrate that 20 per cent of working women in the US are in the perimenopausal and postmenopausal stages of their life cycle. Reports from Harvard Medical School (2009), *The New York Times* (2018) and AARP (American Association of Retired Persons) (2018) indicate that between 40 per cent and 84 per cent of women have reported experiencing physical or psychological changes which have caused personal and professional disruption in their lives.

My mother, who passed away recently, was a college professor and she had an onset of early menopause at the age of 44. She often told me that she had night sweats, hot flushes and was unable to focus at work and take care of my sister and myself. Unfortunately, she was not offered any hormonal replacement therapy to alleviate her symptoms (this was forty-two years ago) and no emotional support, so she resigned her job, which she loved, stayed at home for three years, coping as best as she could with her menopause and went back to working part-time until she retired.

Similar to their British counterparts, American women also lack adequate support at their workplaces during climacteric. Physicians, social scientists and researchers recommend the implementation and adoption of supportive workplace polices and safe places for dialogue about menopause, which can contribute to a better understanding and creation of a non-judgemental and non-discriminatory attitude. According to Dr Chris Bobel, professor and chair of Women's, Gender and Sexuality Studies at the University of Massachusetts in Boston, speaking to MarketWatch, ageism is one of the main reasons for few or non-existent work policies on menopause. In cultures where older people, especially women, are considered dispensable or disposable and are often marginalised, this can translate into an attitude of non-concern for women in the work arena.

Menopause human rights: moving forward

Access to doctors and healthcare providers is crucial for women to navigate challenges during the menopausal years, by providing medical treatment, supplements and lifestyle changes on an individual basis as needed.

In addition, a supportive environment at work is essential, as women spend a significant time at their workplaces. Suggestions made by cross-disciplinary experts include employers hiring staff advocates, making educational material about menopause available and providing access to exercise spaces and healthy food options.

Management experts Professors Kathleen Riach and Gavin Jack from Monash University in Australia also suggest other individualised strategies, such as providing fans for women in their work stations, access to temperature control, less restrictive dress codes and the option to work from home when symptoms become disabling without the fear of being stigmatised. The experts, writing in *The Conversation*, further reiterate that these measures are not just about helping to alleviate symptoms of menopause, but also addressing ageism and showcasing the company's policy that older women employees are as valued as their younger colleagues, both male and female.

Europe has so far been at the forefront of menopause strategies and policies in the workplace. The University of Leicester in the UK has started to run Menopause Cafés on campus and in 2019 instituted online management training on menopause as part of a suite of priority issues in human resource management and staff well-being. It has also established a Menopause Research Network, connecting academics with leaders in the private and public sectors. In this way, the university can be an important player in bringing about a change in the culture and attitudes around menopause in the workplace, so that it is not considered a taboo and employers, irrespective of their size, can be enabled to address menopause in the same manner as pregnancy and childbirth.

In the private sector, the global retailer Marks and Spencer has introduced an online resource called 'Manage your Menopause'. This site features video clips and tips and has been well received by the female workforce. In 2017, E.ON in the UK had the distinction of becoming the first menopause-friendly energy company. As reported on its website, the company has worked on developing guidelines for its managerial staff to make sure they have the appropriate training in providing much-needed support. By introducing the guide, raising awareness and undertaking colleague engagement about this natural phase in a woman's life, E.ON says it hopes to encourage open and honest conversations.

In the US, the Bureau of Labor estimates that by 2024 the workforce of women over 55 will be more than 19.5 million, reinforcing that more

efforts are needed by employers to include policies addressing meno-
pause, to facilitate a better working environment for their employees and
to recruit and retain older women workers. Hollywood celebrities such as
Viola Davis, Gwyneth Paltrow, Taraji P. Henson and Pamela Adlon have
been speaking about the 'taboo topic menopause'. Well-known journalist
Monica Corcoran Harel also revealed in an article for *The Hollywood Reporter*,
'Hollywood's Menopause Problem: The Silence Around It Perpetuates
Silence Among Women', that more than twenty actresses declined her invitation to be interviewed. When comedian Melissa McCarthy enacts the role
of a menopausal, middle-aged romance novelist in miniseries *Nine Perfect
Strangers*, activists are hoping that her dramatic on-screen hot flushes could
spark a dialogue that is long overdue and bring to the table the challenges
faced by millions of women when dealing with menopause. In contrast to
Hollywood's relative reticence, in Silicon Valley, former Microsoft media
director Jill Angelo launched an online clinic in 2019 called Gennev.com,
to offer women personalised health programmes, 'telemedicine' access to
menopause-trained doctors and a discussion forum.

In the past decade there has been a slow but conscious effort globally
to address the issue of menopause on a public platform, with blogs from
Menopause Health Matters and Menopause Goddess to Red Hot Mamas and
My Second Spring that offer advice, counselling and services for women.
The Indian Menopause Society (IMS), which was launched a few years ago,
has a blog to educate women about menopause on its website. It features
articles on menopause for the general public in various languages, demon-
strating the conscious efforts in the past few years to bring the discussion
of menopause into the mainstream of society and to de-medicalise it, as it
is not a disease but a normal physiological occurrence in women. Similarly,
the South African Menopause Society (SAMS), a multi-disciplinary organisation, was established to help women cope with menopause and try to
lead normal lives.

There is a close link between menopause and human rights. Women
have been discriminated against, denied access and marginalised in many
societies at the onset of menopause. This gender-based discrimination and
gendered ageism illustrates that the human rights of these women have
been violated. It is important for all involved – especially for women from
various walks of life globally – to advocate for themselves and other women
who are not in a position to do so, in order to ensure that the necessary

support and safety nets are made available for them to cope with and navigate the important milestone of menopause in their lives.

Making menopause a global priority

Hopefully, as the global community celebrates the seventy-fifth anniversary of the United Nations in 2020, menopause will be included in the discussion of women's issues at the women-oriented meetings, such as the Commission on the Status of Women (CSW). The CSW's annual two-week session considers and promotes important issues pertaining to women, including their well-being. Similar to the sustained efforts and campaigns to include addressing the social discrimination against widows and their rights on the global agenda, menopause needs advocates to make sure it is part of the global conversation. Women can attain a complete state of health as defined by the World Health Organisation when their social well-being is addressed and they can enjoy their human rights to the fullest. This can only be achieved when a support system for menopausal women is made a priority by global stakeholders.

A trained obstetrician and gynaecologist who has practised medicine and public health for the past twenty-eight years, **Dr Padmini Murthy** is Professor and Global Health Director at the New York Medical College School of Health Sciences and Practice. Secretary General of the Medical Women's International Association (MWIA) and Global Health Lead of the American Medical Women's Association (AMWA), she is widely published and has made over 150 presentations on women's and children's health nationally and internationally. Dr Murthy's research interests are women's health and human rights, social determinants of health, and diplomacy and promotion of global health. She has been working to promote safe motherhood and other health initiatives focused on women in India, Malawi and Grenada. Dr Murthy has been the recipient of numerous national and international awards, including the Elizabeth Blackwell Medal for her service to women and the Soujourner Truth Pin, which is given to those women who excel in community service. She is First Vice President of the Global NGO Executive Committee affiliated with Department of Global Communications, United Nations and Chair Elect of the International Health Section of The American Public Health Association.

3

Making Menopause Matter

Diane Danzebrink's compelling account of her own experiences, her menopause advocacy and founding of the groundbreaking #MakeMenopauseMatter campaign are powerful reminders of how menopause awareness is vital for a healthy society.

A few years ago, I hadn't given menopause a second thought. Fast-forward to today and menopause and mental health are pretty much all I think, talk and write about. In the early part of 2012 I was struggling with my health in a way that I never had before. I was really tired and felt washed out all of the time; I was pale, I could almost fall asleep standing up and I just wasn't functioning normally for me. I had zero energy. To be fair, the weather was pretty horrible – typical British winter, cold, grey and wet – but I reassured myself that lots of people felt the same way when the days were long, dark and grey. As winter gave way to spring, however, I felt worse, not better. One of my favourite things to do every day is to walk my dogs, but even that had become a chore. I had started to feel quite anxious and emotional and was finding it increasingly difficult to cope with my normal busy daily life.

Eventually my husband persuaded me to visit the doctor. When I sat in front of her, I explained my symptoms and how long they had been going on. I told her just how tired and lifeless I felt and she suggested running some blood tests. The results were in about a week later and showed that I was very anaemic. I had suffered with very heavy periods, including flooding and clotting, for several years. I had never sought help from the doctor – my mum suffered similarly and I thought it was just part of getting older. When I took the time to look back, I realised that I had actually been struggling for over ten years and most months I would be confined to the house for a couple of days. The doctor explained that my iron level was very low as a result of the regular heavy bleeding; she prescribed some iron tablets and told me to return if I didn't feel better in a few weeks.

I didn't feel better. In fact, I felt worse. More blood tests were run and a few days later my doctor rang me (you always know there is something seriously wrong when your doctor calls you). The doctor explained that my blood results had raised concerns about possible ovarian cancer; my mother had been diagnosed with ovarian cancer some years earlier. Things moved quickly and it wasn't long before I found myself at the hospital having an ultrasound scan which showed that I had complex cysts on both of my ovaries and a large fibroid. I had been convinced that the scan would be clear and I can still remember walking down the corridor hand in hand with my husband, telling him what had been found with the tears streaming down my cheeks. The next stop was more scans followed by an appointment with the gynaecologist.

My scan results and family history were discussed, along with my most recent blood tests, which had caused more concern. The gynaecologist explained that it might be ovarian cancer but that there could be other possibilities; the best option would be for me to have a total abdominal hysterectomy including the removal of both of my ovaries and my cervix. The gynaecologist explained that keyhole surgery, removing just the ovaries, ran the risk of shedding cells, which would be a disaster if cancer was diagnosed. To be honest, when somebody tells you that they think you have ovarian cancer you want the surgery done there and then. The days spent waiting for my hospital admission were the longest of my life.

The morning after my surgery the gynaecologist came to see me to explain that the operation had been longer and more complex than expected, as she had discovered both severe endometriosis (tissue similar to the womb lining growing into other abdominal organs) and adenomyosis (where womb lining breaks through the muscle wall). So that explained all the pelvic and lower back pain that I had been experiencing for so many years. The adhesions caused by endometriosis had made operating very tricky and unfortunately my bladder had been damaged during the operation, hence the attractive bag attached to my leg. The good news was that having seen the growths on my ovaries, she was quietly confident that my surgery had been done, in her words, 'just in time'; lab results would confirm whether or not she was right when they arrived. As I had no control over the results, I focused my attention on getting out of bed and proving to the nurses that I was well enough to go home. On day two I carefully pushed myself to shower, dress and take a short, uncomfortable shuffle past the nurse's station unaided and that afternoon I left the hospital with an appointment to return two weeks later to have my catheter removed.

When the envelope containing the lab results dropped through the letterbox it took me a while to pluck up the courage to open it. When I finally read it, the letter confirmed that no malignancy had been found. As you can imagine, I was enormously relieved and felt very lucky. I wanted to do everything that I could to look after my health and get on with my life.

Before I left the hospital, I was simply told to book an appointment with my GP when I felt up to it to talk about HRT, as there would be no follow-up with the gynaecologist – which I was shocked to hear. Many years earlier my mum had been given an HRT implant following her surgery for ovarian cancer and, being curious, I decided to research what was in her HRT. When I found out that it was derived from horse urine I was horrified and decided there and then that HRT would not be for me in the future. Despite being in surgical menopause, nobody had taken the time to counsel me about all the possible symptoms and long-term health concerns that such a dramatic menopause could cause and I had no idea. I had started to experience hot flushes, but if they were all I had to put up with then I figured that I had been very lucky and I would cope with them.

I found a women's health clinic and decided to visit as soon as I was fit enough. At my first appointment the nutritionist, who was very confident that she could help me manage surgical menopause with supplements, prescribed several herbal remedies and assured me that they would help with my symptoms and look after my long-term health. In the first few weeks after surgery everything was going well and I was even strong enough to attend the London Paralympics. I thought it was all going to be onwards and upwards from there.

A few months after surgery, however, things went very wrong, very quickly. Physically I was doing well, but mentally I was starting to struggle. Initially I noticed that I was becoming increasingly anxious and generally feeling less confident. My sleep pattern had fallen apart and I was spending most nights lying awake, desperate for sleep. Sometimes the fear and anxiety would become so overwhelming that I would need to shake my husband awake to reassure me – really not what he needed, particularly as he had pretty much had to take on the responsibility for everything, including going to work every day, as my mental health deteriorated.

As time went on the anxiety was regularly accompanied by panic attacks. I became less able to focus and concentrate, until eventually any sort of work became completely impossible. By this time, I was leaving the house less and less and was reluctant to see friends, answer the phone or open letters – which I was convinced would only contain bad news. Sometimes I felt so heavy that I just could not get out of bed and on my worst days it would take me several hours to get from the bed to the shower a few feet away.

I had never experienced depression before, but each day felt darker than the last and getting through them was like wading through chest-deep treacle. I was becoming increasingly insecure and irrational but continually refused to see the doctor, as I thought I was going mad and was convinced the only way forward was a lifetime of anti-depressants. Finally, my husband had no choice but to ask my mum to come and stay, as he had become so concerned about my mental health that he was worried what I might do if left alone while he went to work.

My poor mum looked after me during the day and was regularly woken during the night, when I would creep along the landing, crawl into bed with her and just sob my heart out like a child in an effort not to disturb my poor exhausted husband. The future looked bleak to me; I felt useless, hopeless and worthless. I had no idea where the real me had disappeared to; I had lost my joy. I felt sad, frightened and lost. I was unrecognisable. What made all this worse is that I have always been the person that others come to for support and advice. The strong, sensible, level-headed friend who can always be relied upon to apply a healthy dose of common sense and balance to any situation, to help you find a solution to any problem. Somewhere along the line I had become a shadow of the real me and I had no idea how I would ever find her again.

My husband and mum tried so many times to convince me to go back to see the doctor, but I refused repeatedly. I was terrified. I did agree to see the nutritionist again, but as we sat in her office she started to consult books for answers and any hopes I had quickly faded away. I started to surf the internet at stupid o'clock in the morning when I couldn't sleep, to see if anybody was feeling as dreadful and scared as me and I was shocked to find thousands of women saying things like, 'Please help me I think I am going mad, I feel so lost, so alone.'

One day I was so desperate that I rang my GP surgery looking for a support group. It had taken me several hours to pluck up the courage to make the call and I was devastated when the receptionist told me that there was nothing like that. I clearly remember falling in a sobbing heap on to the sofa. That had been my last hope; I could not believe that there was nothing out there for me. When I finally stopped crying, I told my husband just how ludicrous it was that menopause, which would affect so many, was so badly supported and if I ever felt like me again I would make damn sure I changed it.

One morning soon after, I came very close to taking my own life. I had not driven for some time and I still don't remember putting my dogs in the boot of the car or the first part of the drive, but I found myself on a dual carriageway close to my home and decided that I was too much trouble for everyone around me and that it would be better if I was no longer here. I clearly remember the lorry that I was going to put my car into the path of and at the very point of making the manoeuvre one of my dogs started to bark. I was brought sharply back to reality and began to sob and shake violently at the thought of what I had almost done. I don't know how I drove home and I don't remember much about the rest of the day other than telling my husband what I had almost done.

Unbeknown to me, my husband immediately contacted our GP practice and that evening I sat in front of the doctor sobbing through the details of the past few weeks. I was so desperate for help but determined not use the HRT my mum had been given or to take anti-depressants. The doctor explained that I was experiencing such severe symptoms due to my lack of oestrogen, caused by the removal of my ovaries, and only oestrogen could help and no amount of herbs, vitamins and minerals would replace the oestrogen. She went on to tell me about body-identical, plant-derived HRT, which was different from the version my mum had been prescribed. She assured me it was what I needed. I have often heard people speak about having a weight lifted from their shoulders, but I had never experienced it until that moment. The little square plaster-like patch that she prescribed for me to stick on my thigh twice a week made a huge difference very quickly and the world no longer felt like such a dark, scary place, but it wasn't long before relief turned to anger. Looking back at what I had almost done made me wonder how many other women had felt that way due to a lack of the right information and support. It was then that the die was cast for the future; but at that point my own recovery was far from complete.

I went from strength to strength for several months, but I had been doing lots of research and realised that as somebody who had finally been diagnosed with such severe endometriosis, my replacement oestrogen should have been accompanied by replacement progesterone, at least in the first couple of years. It's important to say that progesterone is prescribed alongside oestrogen for women with a womb to protect the womb or endometrial lining. For most women who have had their womb removed, progesterone is not required; but it's important initially if you have had endometriosis. I went back to my GP surgery but the doctor I saw didn't know anything about the research I had read, so referred me to a menopause specialist.

When my appointment to see the menopause specialist finally arrived I was exhausted, as my sleep had fallen apart again, partly due to the horrible heart palpitations that I was experiencing. The doctor listened patiently to why I had been referred to her and pronounced that progesterone was 'a horrible hormone' and she would not prescribe it, but suggested my doctor should prescribe a very small dose of testosterone. To be fair, I had read that testosterone should be considered for women in surgical menopause, but she did nothing to quash my fears about the endometriosis returning without progesterone. I left the hospital in tears; I had waited so long and was sure that this specialist would know why I should have progesterone. I had read so much that clearly indicated oestrogen-only HRT was not appropriate for those who had suffered with severe endometriosis, as it was possible that the oestrogen could stimulate any remaining endometrial tissue. Endometriosis can only be treated with surgery and I wanted to do everything that I could to avoid further surgery. I spoke with my own doctor once again and she insisted that she could not prescribe progesterone, so I decided to take matters into my own hands and booked to see a private menopause specialist. The specialist confirmed that all my research was correct and that I should have been prescribed oestrogen, progesterone and testosterone initially, and that I should have been counselled about this prior to my surgery.

Once I had the right treatment in the right doses and the right support I started to feel like me again. However, I simply could not forget all those women I had come across online, what menopause had almost driven me to do or that if I had not been in the fortunate position to be able to seek advice from a private specialist how I might still be struggling. I began to wonder what I could practically do to change things for women in the future. Many years earlier I had studied counselling but had taken a different career path. I made the decision to go back to studying psychotherapy and menopause, and while I was studying set up the Menopause Support website, aimed at sharing factual, evidence-based information for women and their families.

In November 2015 the very first National Institute for Health and Care Excellence (NICE) menopause guidelines were published and there was quite a lot of press coverage. Having written about my own experience and published it online I was contacted by the BBC and asked to appear on the *Victoria Derbyshire* programme. I had never been on TV, but it was too good an opportunity to discuss something that I passionately felt needed to be talked about more openly. This was my opportunity and I was not going to let it pass by, despite the nerves. A few hours after the programme my inbox was jammed with emails from women sharing heartbreaking experiences of how their undiagnosed and untreated menopause symptoms had affected their lives. It was both shocking and humbling to have complete strangers share such intimate details of their lives in a bid to find the help they so desperately needed.

Studies completed, I decided to specialise in counselling women about menopause in the hope of helping some of those so desperate for help. I also began to receive requests from both TV and radio to speak about the barriers that women faced to being able to access the right help and support, and the wider effects of menopause on mental health, relationships and careers. Life had taken a very unexpected turn, but I was delighted to be able to raise wider awareness. Coming out of the BBC one morning my phone rang and when I answered it the voice at the other end was that of MP Carolyn Harris. She was inviting me to Westminster, to offer her help in raising awareness in parliament of the issues around menopause care and support that she had heard me discussing. I have been to Westminster many times now and

I am very grateful to Carolyn, Rachel Maclean MP and former MP and women's health champion Paula Sherriff for their support in putting menopause on to the parliamentary agenda.

By this time, I was supporting women professionally, speaking publicly and working with MPs, but it still felt as though I was only scratching the surface. So after a lot of thought I decided to set up a private Facebook group called the Menopause Support Network and shortly after a national campaign called #MakeMenopauseMatter. The Facebook group has grown beyond what I ever expected and now, thanks to my amazing team of volunteer moderators, supports 15,000 women. Starting the campaign was a knee-jerk reaction to reading yet another distressing email from a woman who had been failed terribly – to be honest, I had no idea how huge the issue was until I started talking and writing about it – but on this particular night I just decided that I needed to do something bigger. So I sat at my computer, wrote the campaign petition and aims, and pressed the upload button. I really had no idea if anyone would ever sign it, or if anyone would agree with the three aims that I had decided were the most pressing. They are:

1. To ensure mandatory menopause training for all GPs;
2. To have menopause guidance in every workplace;
3. To have menopause included in the new relationships and sex education (RSE) curriculum.

I am absolutely delighted to say that many thousands have now signed the petition since its launch in October 2018. To date in July 2020, we have well over 115,000 signatures and just nine months after launching we achieved the aim of having menopause included in the curriculum, which was incredible, as I had been warned by seasoned campaigners that these things can take many years to achieve and you have to be in it for the long haul. One down, two to go!

If you are wondering why this matters to our society as a whole, I wanted to share some statistics with you, along with some of the very real reasons why menopause awareness and support benefits us all. Menopause matters because three in four women will experience symptoms with one in four describing them as debilitating. In 2018, a survey was commissioned for the BBC, the results showing that 48 per cent of the women between 50 and 55 said that their mental health was affected by their menopause symptoms; 25 per cent said it made them want to stay at home, which corresponds with the one in four who experience debilitating symptoms.

In 2019 the Chartered Institute of Personnel and Development (CIPD) released the results of its survey, which showed that 59 per cent of women between the ages of 45 and 55 said menopause symptoms had a negative impact on them at work. Many had taken sick leave and over 30 per cent felt they couldn't disclose the reason to their manager, as they felt that he or she would not be supportive. In a 2017 survey for the British Menopause Society, 51 per cent of respondents said that their menopause symptoms had affected their sex lives and 38 per cent of partners said that they felt helpless to support their partner.

Menopause is not a women's issue; while it is women who are directly affected, the impact of menopause can affect partners, families, friendships and careers. There is a gaping hole where menopause education and information should exist. Historically, none of us have been formally taught about menopause, which means that when it happens to you or a loved one you probably don't recognise the symptoms as menopause or know what to do to help yourself or somebody else. Menopause has not been talked about openly, which has led to it being stigmatised and often the butt of jokes, due to a lack of understanding.

I find myself in London quite often these days for speaking or presenting engagements. Frequently I jump in a cab at the station and invariably the cab driver will ask me what I am going to be doing at my destination. I often say that I will presenting or doing an interview and the next question is always what about. When I say menopause there is usually a silence, followed by details of how it has affected my driver's wife or partner and their relationship. I can almost guarantee that the conversation will start not with how the hot flushes or night sweats impacted their relationship, but with how the lesser-known psychological symptoms affected them both: the increased anxiety, the mood swings, the irritability, the reduced confidence, the partner no longer wanting to socialise, the feelings of isolation when partners withdraw into themselves, the physical isolation when there is no longer any hugging or kissing and definitely no sex.

What starts as a joke very quickly becomes deadly serious and the conversation turns to how these men wished they had known how to support their partners. I have heard emotional men talk about the breakdown of their marriages; I have been told about affairs that are regretted every single day and about the loss that these men feel. I am always truly honoured that they choose to share these life experiences with me, but it is heartbreaking, as these painful experiences could have been prevented for these men and their partners with a little education at the right time. I've also had two female cab drivers, who were both desperate for more information once they knew what I did.

I regularly teach public menopause workshops and we talk about everything, including the most intimate of symptoms which affect the vulva and vagina. It is shocking how many women are living with urinary incontinence or discomfort of the vulva or vagina and accepting that it is just part of getting older or just getting on with it as they are too embarrassed to discuss it, even with their doctor. These symptoms are treatable and manageable for the vast majority, and let's be absolutely clear that despite what certain advertisers would want you to believe in order to buy their products, urinary incontinence is certainly not normal, nor should it be accepted as such.

The vaginal symptoms of menopause can be both physically and mentally debilitating and can have a drastic effect on quality of life. Vaginal dryness or soreness often leads, quite understandably, to a reluctance to engage in any physical contact whatsoever, and if this is not discussed with a partner it can lead to those feelings of rejection and isolation previously discussed. I was speaking about this at a recent workshop when a woman raised her hand, I thought to ask a question. She didn't have a question; she simply said: 'I wish I had known all this two years ago. I think the information you have just shared could probably have saved my marriage.'

I regularly hear from women who have been told they are too young to be experiencing menopause, or that they are not having hot flushes so it can't be menopause, or that they are stressed and depressed and need antidepressants, or that they should wait until their symptoms get worse before they start treatment for menopause. Many of these women have been backwards and forwards to their doctors many, many times with a host of what seem like unrelated symptoms. I have spoken to women incorrectly diagnosed with irritable bowel syndrome (IBS), fibromyalgia, mental health conditions, the list goes on. So much needless suffering, so many repeat GP appointments wasted and so many secondary referrals made for symptoms that could be simply recognised and managed with the right professional education. Women, their families, GPs and the NHS are paying a very high price for this woeful lack of education.

The costs do not end there. The workplace is also experiencing the cost of a lack of menopause awareness. I regularly go into workplaces as part of my work to deliver menopause awareness and manager training. I can guarantee that after the session there will be a queue of mainly women who want to talk to me. I am always keen to ensure that I speak to everyone, as the ones at the back of the queue hang back for a reason: they are the ones who are usually struggling in the workplace and are only just able to hold back the tears. Many of these women love the work they do and, having sat through the presentation, they suddenly realise why they have been unable to concentrate, or why their anxiety has stopped them being as effective as they usually are, or that their horrifically heavy periods or regular hot flushes are having a devastating effect on their ability to focus and have destroyed their confidence.

A little understanding and compassion and a few simple adjustments can make all the difference and working for an employer actively engaged in raising menopause awareness and making it OK to talk about it at work can have the most dramatic effect. It can make the difference between keeping and losing a valued member of staff. Menopause awareness and support in the workplace is not rocket science and it is a win–win situation for women and their employers.

The mental and emotional impact of menopause should not be underestimated, but nor should the power of being able to help yourself or a loved one. Menopause is often described as a transition ('the process or a period of changing from one state or condition to another', according to the *Oxford Learner's Dictionaries* online). That transition can be very positive when we feel able to take control and plan for the next stage of our lives. My journey to transition was unplanned and much earlier than I expected, and it certainly did not feel positive for a long time; but it has led to me meeting and working with some of the most amazing people, all passionate about improving women's healthcare, and I am deeply thankful to each and every one of them.

It is just common sense to make menopause education and awareness a priority for our healthcare professionals, business leaders and the general public, to avoid the breakdown of relationships and families, costs to our health service and to industry – but most importantly for women's short- and long-term health and well-being.

The truth is very simple: if you are a woman, know a woman or love a woman you need to know about menopause, we must be the generation to #MakeMenopauseMatter.

Diane Danzebrink is a psychotherapist, well-being consultant and menopause expert who works as a therapist in private practice (dianedanzebrink.com) and is the founder of the not-for-profit organisation Menopause Support (menopausesupport.co.uk), which offers menopause education, information, advice and support to the public via telephone consultations, public workshops and a private Facebook community, and menopause awareness training and consultancy to businesses and organisations. In 2018, Diane founded the national #MakeMenopauseMatter campaign, which has already ensured menopause education in the secondary school relationships and sex education (RSE) curriculum and continues to campaign for mandatory menopause education for GPs and better menopause support in the workplace. Regularly interviewed on both TV and radio, she has appeared on ITV, Sky and BBC News, *Lorraine*, *This Morning* and *Good Morning Britain* and both national and regional BBC radio; she has also written about menopause for the *Telegraph* and the *Guardian*.

4

Reflections on a Period of Change

Acclaimed screenwriter **Carol Russell**, whose screen credits include writing for the BAFTA 2020 nominated series *Soon Gone: A Windrush Chronicle* and being part of the BAFTA-winning team behind the *Story of Tracy Beaker*, explores how her own menopause experiences inspired her to champion midlife representation on screen and in life.

I am a story fiend! Ever since I was a little girl, I've loved books. I have learned so much about the world and myself from the books I've read. So, it should be no surprise that I learned about the menopause from a book. My journey began when I was working as an African and Caribbean storyteller. I'd gone to a school in North London and had arrived really early so I parked up near a few shops, one of which was a charity shop with a huge bookshelf outside, and I can never resist browsing through books. That's when I found 'The Book': it was quite thick with a purple cover and the word *Perimenopause* in yellow and underneath, *Changes in Women's Health After 35*. The book called out to me. After all, I was a woman, I was over 35 and besides, I didn't really know anything about menopause except that's when my period would stop. I'd had a love/hate relationship with my period my whole life, so this book about what was going to happen to me next really spoke to me. I flicked through the pages, noting the interesting chapter headings: 'Management of Stress and Depression' and 'Premenstrual Syndrome in Your Transition Years', and that was it – I knew I had to have this book. I looked at the sticker on the front of the book and discovered it was £1.50, so I walked into the shop and handed over my money. When I'd finished working and got myself home, I opened it to the first chapter and began the journey through my perimenopause and menopause that I'm still on today. Throughout this time, it is this book that has helped me every step of the way.

One of the reasons the book called out to me so loudly was because three years before it came into my life, I'd missed two periods on the trot and, a little worried, I decided to go to the doctor. The female doctor I saw ordered a raft of tests, including a hormone test, but she was very clear with me that she didn't think I'd started my menopause. She thought it was stress and she told me not to worry and to go home and have a cup of tea. I did as I was told, and a week later the results came back and it was just as my GP had said – I was fine. The subsequent conversation we had went along the lines of: *You're not in menopause. You're not even close to menopause. Your hormone levels are normal for your age right now. In fact, you can still have babies with no trouble at all. What is going on in your life right now?* As I answered the question, I realised she was right about the stress – I was going through a divorce. So, everything made sense. But now, three years later, I was in a different place and felt that changes were on their way and suddenly I had a companion – The Book.

One of the first things I remember reading was about the changes to memory. That was news to me – unwelcome news. But as well as giving me the problem, the book also gave me the solution: take on new mental challenges. So, I decided to learn Italian and it turned out to be just one of the many benefits of owning the book. One of the other benefits of reading it were the conversations it initiated with my women friends. As I dipped into the book, I shared the various strategies I discovered with my friends. In my friendship group I'm right in the middle – I have friends who are six years older than me, and friends who are six years younger than me. We have had hours of fun in passionate discussions about the strategies I've found in the book, versus things they've tried and tested. The book has also done the rounds in my friendship group; I just got it back recently, and it will be going out again soon. It has been a boon having something that has helped me know, as well as understand, what to expect as I journey through my transition.

During the early years of my perimenopause one of the symptoms I experienced was an extraordinary sensitivity in my body that the book couldn't provide an explanation for, but I love that – I love that it doesn't have all the answers. I've also had the common symptoms: the hot flushes, fragmented sleep, night sweats and irregular periods. As the transition progressed, these maladies were joined by vaginal dryness, reduced stamina, irritability, minor depression, short-term memory loss, difficulty concentrating and mood swings – aka rage, which could be triggered by anything. Still, the melanin in my skin has saved me from the wrinkles – so there's a plus. Of all these symptoms, it's the irregularity of my periods that has caused me the most confusion and has seemed to coincide with the rage. Initially, my periods would disappear for a couple of months, then suddenly – *Hello, I'm back!* – and they'd be around for a while then gone again. This flux reminds me of a friend who told me her story of going for eleven months without a period and then, when she had just thrown away her sanitary products – thinking, *It's done* – back it came! So, I still have products in the bathroom... just in case.

The symptom that's the cause of the most rage is the short-term memory loss – which I affectionately refer to as the 'brain farts'. These lapses infuriate me, especially when my brain fails me in the middle of a sentence and I completely forget what I'm talking about, and even why I'm talking. It's the symptom I've worked hardest to hold at bay. When these lapses first started to occur, I would feel low – I didn't know why they were happening and I was angry that this was happening to me. Throughout my life up until this point, my memory was one of my greatest assets. My memory has been fundamental to my career: I had trained as an actress, a job for which a good memory is a prerequisite; as an international storyteller of African and Caribbean tales my memory was important; as a corporate consultant specialising in story, a lot of public speaking and facilitating workshops called for a good memory. The book has really helped, first by informing me that short-term memory loss is a symptom of menopause, and secondly by suggesting strategies to deal with it as seamlessly as possible. Nevertheless, I went through the five stages of grief, although I think I skipped denial and went straight into rage. I talked with my friends; they listened to me weep, wail and grieve. But once I accepted that this loss was something I was going to have to live with, I realised I had to learn to consciously trust myself and to trust that my memory hadn't completely disappeared, but that it needed some help. So, when a conversation is really important, I record it on my smartphone, which means I can relax and listen and this ironically means I remember more anyway.

As me and my Black women friends have progressed through our transitions, one of the things we have talked about is how to deal with the physical symptoms of the menopause: black cohosh and evening primrose oil for the hot flushes; or yellow yam or soya and other traditional African and Caribbean herbal remedies for general health. Black cohosh I found really useful in the early days; evening primrose oil less so. Soya was good, but yellow yam was better as it helps with hormone replacement, and I think it also helps with the management of my cholesterol levels. However, for me there came a point when food and herbs alone were not enough to keep the physical symptoms at bay, because the night-sweats were waking me up every single night and sometimes several times a night. These fitful nights meant I was often tired the next day, and that triggered the rage because I was afraid I would make mistakes. So, I decided to go see my GP again. When I'd gone before all those years ago with my menopause scare, my GP had been an older woman – probably going through her menopausal transition at the time. This GP was much a younger woman. She was really efficient; she gave me plenty of options and a cancellation meant she was able to give me a double appointment. I decided on hormone patches and soon the hot flushes were gone, and I was able to sleep at night. The patches also helped with the short-term memory loss, but there were trade-offs: trade-offs that I felt were worth living with.

Women's reproductive lives from first periods to menopause were taboo subjects when I was growing up, because my mother was an old-fashioned, old-school Edwardian style parent. She was from that Windrush generation, so health in general wasn't discussed at all. My mother used to send me to the chemist to buy her sanitary towels; she'd send me with a note and money in a bag with instructions to wait until the shop was empty before handing the bag over to the lady behind the counter. The woman would take the bag and replace the note and the money with sanitary towels and give me the change and I would run back home, adhering to my mother's final instruction not to look in the bag. That errand always made me feel like a spy; I enjoyed it as I felt like I was in *Mission: Impossible* or *I Spy*, or *The Man from U.N.C.L.E.* Then one day, when I was about 11, Mum sent me to the chemist and when I got home she called me to my bedroom and took the sanitary towels out of the bag and said, 'When your blood comes, you need to wear this and you need to wear this,' and she gave me the belt and the sanitary towels before clearing one of the drawers in my dressing table and telling me to keep them there. She didn't show me how to use the sanitary towel, so I had no idea what you did with it, or how it was worn.

I was twelve and a half when 'My Blood' came. It was a Sunday and we'd gone to a party as a family the night before and I'd met a boy I really liked. We'd swapped phone numbers written on the back of a fag packet in lipstick and we were going to meet the next day on Wandsworth Bridge. I went to bed excited and woke up the next morning in a bed full of blood and in agony. I'd been brought up a Catholic and, in that moment, I really believed this was God's punishment because I'd met a boy and was therefore a bad girl. I remember lying in the bed in pain and thinking, *Oh God, how am I going to explain this to my Mum?* I didn't know where the blood had come from or what was going on. My Mum finally came into my room to find out why I wasn't up and dressed and going to church, and eventually I showed her the blood. I thought I was in deep trouble, but she just said, 'Right, take your nightie off, and go and have a bath.' When I returned, she'd stripped and remade the bed, laid out my favourite nightie and a sanitary towel, and slipped a hot water bottle in between the sheets, which she told me to put on my stomach for the pain. I was allowed to stay in bed all day. A few days later, once the pain had gone and my period was over, my Mum came and said, 'Right. Now you can get pregnant – DON'T!' That was it. Talking to my cousins about it afterwards, we'd all gone through a version of that experience.

A few years later, the next time we discussed reproduction, my cousin was pregnant and had come to see my Mum because she was afraid to tell my aunt on her own. After my Mum had comforted my cousin and promised to be with her when she told my aunt, she and I waved her off and, as we watched her walk down the road, my mother put her arm around me and said, 'Do NOT get pregnant.'

The journey I'm on now feels very similar to the one I made at the beginning of my reproductive life; it is a journey marked by anger and fear. Talking with my women friends, hearing their stories and thoughts about their experiences of starting and ending menstruation has helped me understand my own journey more. I suspect the rage I felt at the beginning of my childbearing years was also to do with the fact that as a girl my life was mapped out for me by the society in which I lived. Everything my mother did and said to me made me aware that my days of climbing trees, riding bikes, jumping from 10ft walls and rolling like I'd leapt from a plane in a parachute, playing football, running until I was tired and spinning in the sunshine until I was dizzy, would soon be over. The rage I felt as a girl on the brink of young womanhood was actually grief for my loss of freedom. As I approached puberty, I was expected to do more and more in the house: cooking and cleaning, washing and ironing clothes, looking after my little brother – women's work as it was called then. So, it was a slow and steady build to the loss of my freedom rather than a sudden shift. Though the start of my period was a milestone because my life really did change after that. My mother began to watch me like a hawk, and I realise now that her fear wasn't of me, but for me. She knew the traps that lay ahead for me, to tie me to the home. She understood the predators who lay in wait and the pain and loneliness that come with being a lone parent. She didn't want that for me. My mother is proud of me and all I've achieved. She's never said it to me, but my brother told me that when I was working as an actress, my mother would always have in her handbag a copy of the programme of whatever play I was appearing in and whenever she met with any of our family or her friends and they asked after me, she would whip that programme out and regale them with tales of my successes.

Recently I have been reflecting on the fact that when Africans were enslaved and taken to the Americas, a woman was expected to work every bit as hard as a man – even when said woman was pregnant. As women we were 'valued' not only as 'machines' that could be forced to labour and make value out of cotton or sugar cane, or whatever task we performed from which money could be made, but also for the lives we carried and brought into the world. And what has haunted me is discovering from Marcus Rediker's *The Slave Ship* that enslaved African women didn't have periods for up to two years after the trauma of their kidnap and transportation. If we made it to menopause in that society, we were, of course, viewed as less valuable because we were no longer providing 'free' labourers. Plus, we were no longer as profitable in the field as we could no longer work as hard. The older we got, the less value we had. If we made it to as old as 70, we were tasked with looking after the children that were seen as too young to work – the under 4-year-olds.

So, I have come full circle. As the reproductive hormones ebb from my body, I suspect the rage I feel as I come to the end of my child-bearing years is again grief. This time I am grieving for the life I haven't been allowed to live as a woman, especially a woman of African descent. This is coupled with the knowledge that at this time in my life, society doesn't expect me to want to achieve the dreams that have been deferred by my womanhood and my African descent, but instead it would prefer me to take a step back and allow the young to have their turn. But I am one of those who believes there is enough to go around, and that no one has to lose so another can gain. So, as I have done all my life, I will push forward with making my dreams come true because, right now, I believe I can.

As a menopausal woman, the closest I get to seeing myself in popular culture is in African American shows, be they drama or reality TV shows. If menopausal women are seen by popular culture at all, they are frequently seen as figures of fun; their main characteristics are the usual tropes of hot flushes, emotional volatility and frigidity. It's very, very unusual to see a menopausal woman portrayed in a fully rounded way, as a woman who is more than a slave to her hormonal surges.

I remember the first time I saw *The Golden Girls* in the late 1980s and I've enjoyed watching it again recently, especially now that I am firmly in that demographic. The portrayal of women over 50 in the show was so beautifully varied and nuanced. There was not a single frigid woman in the lot. I particularly loved the character of Blanche Devereaux, it was so good see a woman in her fifties portrayed as sensual and sexual, and completely unashamed of her libido. At the time she reminded me, and a number of my friends, of the 'Aunties' – either familial or honorific – who filled all our lives. The Aunty who was bawdy; the Aunty who didn't allow herself to be defined by society, who drank and smoked and danced libidinously. The Aunty, who in my case was my mother's best friend, was the person who shook my mother loose and made her snort as she flung her head back and laughed with her whole body. The Aunty who was a woman with her whole chest, whether she was perimenopausal, menopausal or postmenopausal. Those *Golden Girls* set the bar for the portrayal of menopausal women really high. At the moment on UK television, Sally Wainwright, creator of *Last Tango in Halifax* and *Happy Valley*, is the only writer I can think of who has put the menopausal and postmenopausal woman right at the centre of her dramas. I think this lack of representation is probably because very few women get to write for TV, and certainly very few menopausal women do.

Another reminder of my 'Aunties' comes not from the screen but via the African American artist Faith Ringgold, who also reminds me of myself. In 2019, I went to what I believe was her first exhibition in the UK at the Serpentine Gallery, London. I'd never been there before but I'd previously seen one of her paintings in the Museum of Modern Art (MoMA) in New York. The painting was *American People Series #20: Die* (1967) – it arrested me. People bumped past me as I stood staring at it. It reminded me of Picasso's *Guernica*. It was acquired by MoMA in 2016; the irony of the fact that a painting created in the middle of the Civil Rights Movement was purchased in the midst of Black Lives Matter protests is not lost on me. Faith Ringgold was an activist in her work and in her life. In 1968 she co-founded Ad Hoc Women's Art Committee and went on to protest a major modernist exhibition at the Whitney Museum of American Art as it didn't feature work by any women or any African American artists. And though she was rarely exhibited at major exhibitions she continued to work: she painted; she quilted; she wrote books; she filled warehouses with her pieces when no one would buy them. Years later, here I was, standing in the Serpentine Gallery feeding my mind and my spirit – watching a documentary about her, being emboldened by her story, returning to the gallery to feed again at the table groaning under the weight of her form-breaking creativity as she taught and teaches me by example. One piece, *Change 2: Faith Ringgold's More Than 100 Pounds Weight Loss Performance Story Quilt*, held my gaze for 20 minutes. The centrepiece is a painting on cloth of a thin woman, hand on hips, laughing. Behind her is her shadow – a woman twice her size. Around the edge of this painting are 10 quilted squares, eight with a photograph of her printed on cloth telling the story of why she gained the weight in the first place. The piece was created in 1988 and she was in the middle of her menopause. Many of the quilts in the exhibition were created as Ringgold transitioned. That fact made me smile as I stood taking in every inch of that quilt. I was inspired by her indomitable spirit to continue creating and if the mainstream doesn't want to produce my work, or that of other women of African descent over 50, I'm inventive and will find ways for it to be seen.

From the beginning of my career, my work has fused both creativity and activism. I lived in Jamaica and attended the Edna Manley College of the Visual and Performing Arts, then called the Jamaica School of Drama, at a time when we were encouraged to look at art as a medium for community change. My very first paid job in the theatre sector was as a stage manager with the revolutionary theatre collective, Sistren. Their work explores the intersections between the patriarchal oppression of women, racism and social class. This group of fifteen women ranged from those in their early twenties to those in their early sixties. It was a joy working with them, seeing how they brought their experiences together and made art with them – art that touched everyone who saw it. Their influence, that fusion of social commentary and Caribbean folk culture, informs every aspect of my artistic work to this day.

Most recently I have been working on a theatre project, *Raised Voices*, which aims to recover and amplify the voices and vision of women playwrights of African heritage over 45. It's won an RSL Literature Matters Award, which is so exciting. My experience of being a woman of African Caribbean descent in Britain is one of erasure. Talking to my younger playwrighting peers I've realised that they don't know very much about what we were doing before them. Our work has disappeared, and in many of the art forms there are few to no Black women over 50. The project opens a conversation about whether this demographic is being under-commissioned, under-programmed and, as an audience, under-served. I aim to change that one arena at a time. For me, it's about giving voice or, more accurately, creating a space for that voice to be heard. My current ambition is to work with women exploring their creativity as they make their transition, allowing them to tell their stories in a way that is cathartic and artistic.

I was 51 when I set up my company, Fresh Voices, with the aim of amplifying the voices of writers of African and Asian descent – South and East. I'd been exploring how I could make a difference to the lack of those voices on television. Working with the decision-makers in the industry, I organised script readings at BAFTA; Meet the Commissioners events with ITV; Boot Camp programmes – created for, and delivered in conjunction with, the London Film School – where screenwriters had the opportunity to work with industry professionals to write original pilot scripts for series. I am really proud to have been a part of bringing writers of African and Asian descent to the attention of an industry I love as I journeyed through my transition.

My mother's generation called the menopause, 'The Change'. The Book, which has been my constant companion on this journey, refers to it as a 'transition': another word for change which resonates for me. This period of my life has been one of reflection and change, and as I write we are in the middle of the COVID-19 pandemic which also affords time for reflection and requires a change in how we live and work. The change I've been through informs the change I, along with the rest of the world, must go through now. After what I've been through, I feel like I've got a head start.

Carol Russell's screenplay, *House of Usher*, was one of six short films made by Crucial Productions for the BBC. She was the principal script-writer for two series of *Comin' Atcha*, starring pop group Cleopatra, for ITV. Her monologue, *Horns of a Dilemma*, was broadcast on BBC Radio 4's *Woman's Hour*. She was one of the BAFTA-nominated team of adapters of Jacqueline Wilson's *The Story of Tracy Beaker*. Carol was also one of fifteen writers chosen for the inaugural MediaXchange Advanced Writing for TV Drama programme 2017/2018, and was one of twenty writers chosen from around Europe for the inaugural Series Mania Writers Campus 2018. She has work in development with three produc-tion companies, including GreenAcre Films where she is working on two drama series, *Dark Justice* and *What Happened at Number 4?* Carol wrote one of the multi-award-winning drama series, *Soon Gone: A Windrush Chronicle*, celebrating the 70th anniversary of *The Windrush*, broadcast on BBC Four in 2019, which has now been nominated for a BAFTA 2020. She was longlisted for Thousand Films/Sid Gentle Films screenwriting competition. Carol is currently writing two episodes of the ninth series of *Stone* for BBC Radio 4, and has been accepted on the Criterion Theatre New Writing programme.

5

From Menarche to Menopause: A Mother's Journey

Sophia Tzeng, entrepreneur and non-profit executive, reflects upon the periodicity of her life as she charts the journey from her first period through to menopause and how her own experiences have helped shape her conversations with her daughters, who include Nadya Okamoto – founder of Period. The Menstrual Movement.

Menarche, 1984

My favourite colour was pink, and my favourite pair of trousers were two shades of it, in alternating stripes of bright rose and neon cotton candy. Crisply creased and cuffed at ankle, I belted them high at the waist with a shiny red strap cinched with a faux gold buckle. I wore these along with my favourite shirt, a blue and grey plaid 1980s mish-mosh with too-short sleeves, buttoned all the way to the top and tucked tightly. The outfit made me as proud as any 10-year-old girl might be in her first 'grown-up' outfit, culled together at a bargain store on the outskirts of a sleepy, one-factory town bordering a vast expanse of rural farmland.

'You're a woman now!' my mother yelped over Saturday afternoon crowds at the discount store, the day I discovered those precious trousers. Her high voice cut through the twangy chatter of dozens of fair-haired, feathered and bouffanted matrons rifling through the sale section, over the scrape and clatter of metal-and-plastic hangers heavy with garments being pushed, pulled, examined and replaced on bright chrome racks. 'Only 10 years old!' my mother announced to no one in particular '... and now with period!'

... with period. It had appeared that summer, days shy of my tenth birthday in the form of concentric brown spots, mysterious stains on the pale yellow of a pair of favourite underwear. In the short span of a few months, I had sprouted taller than my mother and teacher at the time, scarring my back and legs with stretch marks and rendering most of my clothes uncomfortably tight.

My parents were at work and my brother must have been away, for I remember hopping from the bathroom, trousers and underwear hanging at the ankles, dodging stacks of paper and piles of clothes and books to find the rotary phone. From the laboratory where she worked, my mother's voice hushed to a low whisper. 'You're only 9,' she repeated a few times, though I had just turned 10, and then she instructed me to bunch toilet paper, place it between my legs and watch TV until she came home.

How lucky I was, she proclaimed that night, for she at 16 had no one tell her what 'it' was when she got it – not her mother nor aunts nor five older sisters nor sisters-in-law, nor any of her cousins or friends. It was *dirty*, she hissed, opening the middle drawer of her heavy mahogany dresser to indicate a stash of thick menstrual pads that looked like blocks of Styrofoam, hidden beneath stray socks and crumpled tights. *Expensive*, she warned, and in the bathroom showed me how to spin makeshift wads of toilet paper and add orphan socks to make one disposable pad last for a whole cycle's duration.

That weekend, as I packed my prized red suitcase to visit cousins, my father approached and stood awkwardly by, watching as I self-consciously tested which worked better: layering nightgown, stuffed animal and tin full of hair ties, or the other way around? He cleared his throat.

'So. Phi. Yah,' he declared, three sentences unto themselves. 'Moh-mee said you have men-stru-a-tion. Is that cor-rect?' He clipped his words and phrases ponderously, as if repeating after his English language cassette or speaking to his students or fellow professors. This was not the familiar father who tossed me high in the air or comforted me through nightmares and thunderstorms, who perched me on his shoulders whenever a vicious-looking dog approached.

I stopped moving, and nodded into my chest.

'Good,' he said, and went away, never again mentioning the subject. Looking back, I recognise that as the moment when familiar niceties abruptly ceased. All I knew was that it had something to do with being no longer a girl, but now a woman.

Despite pleas regarding my imminent death from discomfort or embarrassment, I was not allowed to stay at home from school when the bleeding began again. Instead, I proceeded to the bus stop, and gingerly made my way to an empty padded seat on the school bus, grateful for its dark forest green colour and vinyl surface, off which a leak could be hidden or quickly wiped. I suppressed the urge to exclaim at every sudden surge of flow with the many bumps and turns, and moved with slow, shuffling steps to the classroom. I refused to budge to sharpen a pencil or retrieve a worksheet, mortified by the involuntary eruptions that spewed, heavy between the legs, threatening to overflow.

When called to lead the girls' bathroom line-up, as the tallest girl in the class, I froze and steadily stood, and saw with horror a fresh crimson stain in my yellow bucket seat. I pushed the chair under the desk and moved sideways, back to the wall. I took my place on the girls' side of the doorway alongside the oldest boy by three years. Tough and hunched, with preternatural grizzle and pink face-scars from frequent fights, he had never so much as acknowledged me before. As we waited, he nudged my elbow and pointed to my backside. 'There's blood on your pants,' he said, and shrugged.

Menstruation, 1996

Ageing into middle school, my body bulged, rendering me suddenly defenceless against the stares of boys on the basketball court or the leers of men in grocery stores and shopping malls, on sidewalks and even while standing in line with my mother at the credit union. 'Ten? She looks eighteen!' one said, standing too close as his eyes appraised my burgeoning body. I took to wearing thick sweaters with shirts buttoned up to the chin, chunky jackets even in summer, long slacks that dragged on floors and glasses so thick and vast they swallowed my face, bugging my eyes out and warping the ground. I took to wearing my father's and brother's clothes and shaved half my head. Even as I shed glasses for contact lenses going into high school, and contemporised my fashion, I dressed in boxy khakis slung low on the waist, with loose plaid shirts obfuscating waist and curves. I was in no way ready for the physical prominence and attention of a womanly figure, in addition to already sticking out with my jet-black hair, Asian eyes, and awkwardness as a target for jabs from students and teachers alike.

There is no such thing as gender difference, I avowed each month, as my mother lay bedridden, moaning. 'How heavy periods are, especially after childbirth!' she exclaimed each time. It is only recently, with my own daughters' experiences, that doctors have confirmed to me that our line of women have extraordinarily heavy menses, and I learned later that my mother suffered from other medical complaints that exacerbated the experience, but back then none of us knew that. My father would simply mutter about how weak women were, how emotional, hysterical and irrational – I needed to learn to simply 'be a man', he'd say, and I'd lower my voice and agree. I vowed never to let womanhood, as he defined it, define me.

Starting at 13 and for the next thirty and more years, I pulled regular all-nighters, punishing the body for its feminity. I descended to our scarcely lit, cinderblock basement to do aerobics on grimy floors by videotape while everyone slept. I worked to remove curves, find flatness, and develop angles, repeating movements until muscles tore and the body broke, even and especially during my period. Every cramp and discomfort, I met with ten push-ups, and when the sun rose, I sprinted the 4.6 mile flat loop encircling the staid suburban neighbourhood in which we lived. I strained my voice so much aiming for masculine bass that I lost it every few weeks, reduced to a hoarse whisper. Mind over matter. Spirit over flesh. I poured perspiration into my vast sense of lack driven by the desperate desire to feel fully human, which meant one had to be male.

Maturation into menstruating womanhood meant doing what many women of my generation did: suppress and oppress any aspect of my experience that did not comply with the mainstream – that is to say, the traditional male perspective. Television shows offered hypersexualised characters, pretty pin-ups ranging from vacuous objects of desire to sisters who wished they were, and mothers who used to be. Even family shows communicated that the chief value of a woman resided in her attractiveness and her capacity to serve that dominant gaze with its infantile needs.

As a young and impressionable girl, I retreated to available literature, classics like Louisa May Alcott's treacly *Little Women* and *Rose in Bloom*, and a threadbare, used library copy of a book I put myself to sleep by every night, completing it at least twenty times before finally learning its title my senior year, when it was assigned for English class: Jane Austen's *Pride and Prejudice*. Rereading all of these books recently, I grasp the profound impact each made regarding how I internalised what goodness and good taste meant. I inherited from these books – and the lived experience in a Western culture derived from them – a controlled, constricted model of womanhood that is subservient to manhood, whose chief rebellion lay in wit, words, and outclassing others through intelligence and prudence, with recognition found through one's having a 'pleasant figure' and an alliance with an older empowered white man.

And, of course, in none of these movies or books was the word 'period' ever mentioned, or 'menstruation'. Rather, a good woman is immaculate and closely clad in whatever the times allowed us with respect to bosoms and ample curves, with particular portrayals of femininity defined by skirts and flowers, shades of rose, and heels that hobble. She detests dirt and faints at the sight of blood, which she presumably does not experience monthly, daily for a week – a bloody 25 per cent of her human existence during her menstrual years!

During those precious formative years, I completely internalised the fiction that my female body was somehow lacking. My anti-woman choices freed me from the entrapment, I thought, of serving the success and pleasure of men. This most damaging form of self-abuse was inflicted by myself upon myself until I fully absorbed at the core how very worthless I was as a woman, a menstruator, and a human experiencing feelings, sensitivity and emotional variegation at all, especially menstruation. By the time it came time to graduate from college and pick a pathway, a career, or at least a job, I found myself frozen in nihilism, unable to advance in any defined direction save for one: the one that harkened me to about-face, retreat, and venture backwards into the undiscovered territory of my inner nature and nature at large.

Against the advice of mentors, professors and friends, the year I graduated from college, I moved to an uninhabited ancient cabin on property my parents had purchased fifteen years before in a forlorn, economically depressed area of Indiana, two hours south of Indianapolis. The place was far off the interstate, bordering 600 acres of state forest, 20 miles through undulating state roads and another 6 miles down a dirt track through dense and scarcely populated deciduous forest.

Reared in suburban homes and apartment buildings, with thin skin and a rabid imagination born of too much time and cloistering, I was ill equipped to be a 'woman of the woods' in the rugged shoot-to-eat sense. I barely knew how to read a compass, and while I had purchased a set of plastic-backed Audobon guides, I could not distinguish between the myriad plants and trees, the flowers and leaves, nor name what fauna inhabited the woods, from the million bugs with their various shapes and wing-sounds to the cacophony of birds at the beginning and end of each forest day.

My ignorance positioned me to enter the woods the way a scientist plunges into an undiscovered abyss, or an anthropologist enters an untouched culture: every single experience and thing I encountered felt artefactual, a representative of a greater system ripe for fruitful observation. In time, the daily walks, quietude of mind, and alert listening in the present tense helped me discern the minutest of interactions and relationships between each thing: the one-sided growth on a tree showed the impact of momentary sun through the high canopy. Density of brush indicated newer clearing, and barely flattened grass, a recent resting place for mother doe and fawn. A proliferation of insects signalled leavings of creatures, or the creature itself, newly demised. And then there was myself, my own body, which without anyone else about became its own forest, landscape and experience, itself the miraculous result of aeons of process and, more recently, thousands of years' evolution on the Asian continent and hundreds of years' refinement in a small village south of current Taipei, where thirteen generations of the ethnic Hakka people evolved in what would now be considered rural poverty, farming with water buffalo, balancing harvests on bamboo poles, and developing habits, language, a body of culture and bodies that best survived in the richness of that lush landscape where my parents met. Their transplantation to America resulted in this fleshly inhabitation that was me, born here but with DNA harkening to the ancients and yet here in real time, playing forth for me to feel and record.

In the woods, I noticed that my body waxed and waned to the phases of the moon – bloating and weightiness turned to tenderness and enervation over the course of the lunar month as a point of regular fact. The day prior to each cycle, I might break into weeping on an innocuous walk, overburdened with the weight of the world, feeling alone and helpless to affect anything – I might seek particularities to eat, or positions for sleeping to address a certain sort of lower backache and heartpain. While on my period, as I trudged the woods with pads and wads of toilet paper in place, I felt the natural world respond to me differently, and I myself responded to the world with more exquisite sensitivity. With senses of acceptance and annoyance heightened, events like the sound of the breeze crescendo-ing through trees, or the progressive emergence of evening stars into the dark purple backdrop of an unlit, uncluttered night sky, and the appearance of the thick Milky Way, dividing the universe, interrupted now and again by a bat or owl traversing overhead, brought me to a sense of acute being and also not-being amidst a greater flow of life, undivided from and interwoven with time.

In the woods, I connected with myself as a mammal in a decidedly female body; as a woman walking with the cycles of the moon, and the turning of the earth, harbouring a womb that filled with anticipation and imminence, and emptied with grief and despair. Stripped of social dictates, without a television, with clocks taken down, over the weeks and months, I felt myself becoming a sentient human being capable of absorbing and reflecting upon life at first hand, as opposed to its being filtered, interpreted and imposed. I grew to know a meta-version of myself as a form of consciousness that fully grasps without having to understand and articulate the elegance and interconnectedness of existence beyond the boundaries of space, time and being. In that place, removed from social impression or construction, the experience of menstruation and womanhood felt like a natural event, like a thunderstorm or spring or icy still winter morning that one lives through and learns from, that causes the body pains and decided inclinations, and that flows with permanent impermanence and periodicity, like each season, having a beginning, middle and end, which then comes again.

Maternity, 1998

One gains wisdom reflecting in nature, but not 'street smarts'. Very soon after leaving the woods, I found myself inadvertently pregnant and unhappily married, installed in law school and living in New York City. My apartment's outer windows faced the castle-like fortress of Columbia College's east wall on Amsterdam Avenue, and its grimy inner windows opened to an alleyway webbed by fire escapes and soot-blackened brick on all sides, stretching up to a very slim sliver of sky. Bereft of nature, with tall buildings and bright lights blotting out the sky and stars, I was myself also without a period, and instead a womb swollen with a quickly growing baby. Racked by nausea, awakened to the extraordinary experience of growing a life within, I surrendered my sense of selfhood at that young age to the being that was overtaking.

When Nadya was born, she became my forest and my trees, and together we created, over her first three years, a world of our own within that little apartment, and then within the city, block by block. With every creative input my imagination could provide on scant income and time, over the next seven-year period, between three more pregnancies, two births, four continents, and nursing each child for nearly two and a half years, I had few periods. My body cycled no longer with the moon every month, but instead racheted between stops dictated by the immediate demands of my moon-faced children and their development, discipline, feeding and survival, overlaid by law school then lawyering, then running a business and non-profits and whatever it took to make a family income. In short, my body became the city environment in which I lived, shaped by the demands of a marketplace ill-attuned to the moon.

Over the years, each girl has matured into menarche with their own stories and remembrances, anxieties and elations, which we have shared openly as well as in quiet reflection. Nadya, my eldest, who is now the age I was when she was born, turned one of our challenging phases into a cause she and her team call the 'menstrual movement', and is succeeding in raising awareness of women's natural needs, shaping legislation, global culture and business practices to fit the reality of being a woman.

Menopause, 2020+

Like many people in my generation, reared at a time when 'menstruation' was unmentionable, I can't recall anything ever said to me about the other

M-word either: menopause. It's possible my mother or aunts may have brought it up, the way I do with my daughters, and if they did, I likely dismissed it the way my daughters now do with me, as if I were droning on about retirement plans and hip replacements. In reflection, I now understand that the fact of menopause, like the experience of menstruation, likely deeply defined my family life and relationship with my mother: I was a late baby, so my adolescent and teen years coincided with her perimenopause and menopause years. To this day, I tend to identify my mother by her sacrifice and her pains, expressed volubly over the years, an accumulation of wounds recounted in a harsh litany.

'*Bu de liao!*' my mother would cry, on entering a car-turned-oven in the rabidly hot Indiana heat, or running from stockroom to steaming kitchen, arms full of supplies, or sitting on a stool, three fans blowing at her while she chopped, the air-conditioning blasting on full and the talk shows droning on the television beside her workstation. *Unbearable*, it means. She invariably used it to express her reaction to the heat, as she ran hot and likely ran hotter experiencing the felt heat of menopause. It also spoke to a deeper anguish, the *unbearability* of the life she endured as a brilliant, outspoken woman and immigrant in the 1970s and '80s, shouldering household labours and childrearing as the wife, sister and daughter of traditionalist Chinese Americans from Taiwan; fighting for credit and respect as a biochemist in a male-dominated medical school until she was pushed out to round out her career the only way generations of Chinese in America were allowed: by running a fast-food restaurant.

My mother never complained about her roles, never acknowledged racism or any other factors – like menopause, hot flashes, and being sensitive and emotional – that influenced her decision to leave cancer research to chop cabbage or, as she would say, make cash for colleges. When I was very young, she openly strove to be the next Madame Curie, and worked in the laboratory on the cure for ovarian cancer and other women's issues, such as uncovering the chemical nature of why wombs contract when they do. I later learned that she associated with people like Dr Hans Adolf Krebs, who discovered a key function of metabolism, for which he won the Nobel Prize. By the time I came of age, she was the owner, proprietor, manager, cook, supply clerk, janitor and assistant at her own restaurant on the edge of a movie megaplex parking lot, where she worked fourteen- to twenty-hour days, every day except Christmas and New Year, smelling of egg rolls and pork grease from early each morning until long past midnight. She worked tirelessly and relentlessly until well past 50, even after she slipped and fell one evening at the age of 55, breaking seven ribs and deeply bruising her hip. Just two hours away, living in the woods at the time, I returned immediately to find her at the restaurant, wincing through excruciating pain, perched on a chair clutching ice to her chest and breathing shallowly, directing my father and youngest brother in keeping operations running, and cash coming in. As an adolescent, I had been chided and derided for my own pains, which conditioned me to condemn my mother and all women for theirs. But by this point, the woods had conditioned me out of being that woman who tolerated the fact that her sensibilities and suffering should be seen as taboo, as weakness and as a source of shame and subservience, and we went straight to the emergency room.

Nevertheless, conditioning is strong and so I enter menopause with the default instinct to simply ignore every felt pain and angst as an inconvenience. I still forcibly 'adult' myself into making time and reflective space to check in with how the body feels, and to be open to feeling and exploring whatever it brings up. It is still a task that feels unnatural to a disposition trained entirely to ignore itself.

With my daughters, when I mention menopause or other aches of ageing, their eyes glaze over, as mine once did those decades ago. Within a sentence, they have picked up their phones or turned to each other, connecting about things that matter more to them. While many things pass from generation to generation, the experience of womanhood has also been transformed by our fast-changing mores and technology, and the rapid cultural adaptation from my parents' generation to my own and my daughters'. For example, all of my daughters started the pill very early, prescribed by doctors to manage anxiety and panic attacks from adverse early childhood experiences, as well as our family's heavy menses – and this resulted in completely stopping their periods. Recently, with the COVID-19 quarantine, my daughters went off all non-essential medication, and for the first time were flattened on the couch, moaning and reeling with sudden sensitivities wrought by the hormonal cocktails ravaging their menstruating systems. My daughters feel hot, and swell up. Their wombs ache, and limbs feel disjointed. They have deep bursts of sadness and longing, followed by release and exuberant outpourings of freedom and energy. Suddenly their olfactory systems are sensitised and they become critical of every aspect of the food they eat. Textures overwhelm. 'I can't take this, Mom, I'm going back on the pill or die!' they each declare in turn. And I nod. I empathise, with bittersweet understanding.

I suggest to my daughters that perhaps the experience of menstruation to menopause is an important one, where our history lives in us, a composite of what has evolved in women's bodies over millions of years to prepare us for the physical experience of being successfully pregnant, with the consequent birthing, nursing and caregiving. Perhaps the exquisite sensitivity and powerful communication from our bodies is why my grandmothers, in a place without modern medicine, during a time of high infant mortality and physical hardship, successfully birthed eight and ten children, respectively, without losing a single one – even until they were nearly 50 years old. Perhaps menstruation, PMS and the cycle of the body is an important experience to have, perhaps even a priceless one, for learning physical resilience, as well as caretaking and empathy, attentiveness to emotion and attunedness to the body in a world where schooling, social convention, the marketplace and our modern life tend to orient towards individuality and autonomy, rationality and independence. A world where 'free will' is at the centre, is one that does not anticipate that another being or body might be entirely dependent upon us. So perhaps we should be asking why medicate to adjust to the world, why not redesign the world to adjust to our rightful physical experience?

By this point, my daughters have long left the conversation. I know they hear the hollow of my words, the syllables and consonants within the passionate pronunciations of a now-matronly mother, facing mortality at the end of a biological window they are only at the beginning of. Menarche, Menstruation, Maternity, Motherhood, Menopause and Mortality – all M-words, once upon a time and still in certain circles. To my progressive, supported daughters, they are inconvenient artefacts of our oppressive collective past, when we were more inhibited by biology and constrained by outdated mores that subjugated us to the masculine other. To them, these anachronisms are at most just labels, phases of a woman's life that are increasingly optional at a time when menopause is less a biological, social experience than the latter phase of contemporary life requiring scientific, psychological and practical management to lessen its effects. They scroll and self-snap on their phones, or chat among themselves, as I return to reflection on the preciousness of life and its lessons, and wondering what preparation might be appropriate for becoming no longer privy to a body engaged in the lunar cycles of bending, building and yielding. How will I embrace a life whose purpose can be bent fully and without impediment towards other aims – that I may myself totally decide? Perhaps less mother-hood and moon, and more the constancy of menopause and sun.

Sophia Tzeng is a facilitator and executive strategist for ASCETA, a consultancy that helps non-profit and social impact leaders and teams find their way forward through transformative, inclusive and impactful strategic design. A former corporate attorney, entrepreneur, non-profit executive and professor of business management and collaborative design, Sophia has served on non-profit boards including Period. The Menstrual Movement. She is the mother of three daughters: social entre-preneur, influencer, author and Period. founder Nadya Okamoto; social justice artist and activist Ameya Marie Okamoto; and high school student and aspiring soprano Issa Okamoto. The daughter of immigrants from a long lineage of Hakka people of the Taoyuan region of Taiwan, Sophia was born and raised in the American Midwest, has lived in New York City, Belgium, Alaska and the South Pacific, and now resides in Portland, Oregon, where she is learning to garden during quarantine surrounded by her family and a new pitbull-spaniel puppy, Romeo Blue. Her prior publications include an essay in *Real Simple* and a self-published poetry chapbook, *19 Pulses*.

6

Pakistan: Where There Are No Words

Shad Begum, recipient of the International Women of Courage Award for her pioneering work in Pakistan, asks how women can begin to have a conversation about something for which there is no word, in places where women's health has been underprioritised for so long.

Growing into womanhood in Pakistan

Before I can explore what the menopause means for women in Pakistan, I need to explain to you what it means to be a woman in Pakistan. In particular, what it means to be a Pashtun woman, as that is my own cultural background and that of the region where I have talked to other women about their understanding of menopause.

Dir, located in the foothills of the Himalayas, is my hometown. Dir was Pakistan's princely state, ruled by a cruel Nawab until its merger into Pakistan in 1969. Our prince was completely against the development of his community. I remember my father quoting the Nawab's era: 'Nawab will not even allow people to whitewash their houses or wear white clothes, as white is the colour of honour and only the prince deserves the right to use and wear white, not his people.' At the time of my birth, only 6 per cent of boys and 1 per cent of girls received any schooling at all. In 1996, Dir was split into two districts, Lower Dir and Upper Dir, for administrative purposes.

I am lucky to have been born in a family that was enlightened. After the merger into Pakistan, my late uncle Dr Dost Muhammad and my father Dr Noor Muhammad, by profession a doctor of pharmacy, founded a welfare organisation called Idara Khidmat-e-Khalq (IKK) to assist the local communities to manage their problems. After the sudden death of my uncle in a road accident, my father started leading IKK. While I was growing up, I was very close to my father and would spend much of my time with him, joining him in his social activities and in his clinic after school. He would always take me to social and political gatherings, where I would listen and talk to men about our area's social and political problems. Most of them called me the 'Benazir of Dir', in reference to Benazir Bhutto, who later became the first woman prime minister of Pakistan. I had no problem with that!

When I turned 16, my father asked me to stop coming with him; he said that now I was a young woman, my place was at home. I was shocked and not happy with this. My mother tried to console me, saying how, due to the cultural barriers, it was difficult for my father to take me along with him now. I was upset and so was my father; he could see that I was sad. He finally sorted out a way for me to remain engaged. He asked me to help him reach out to more women in our community, as his organisation was having difficulty doing this.

I joined as a volunteer, and along with me came the wives and daughters of my father's colleagues. Collectively, the new entrants – us women – started connecting with the women of our community, supporting them in resolving the issues they faced. These mainly related to health, education, employment, domestic violence and so-called 'honour killing'. During my time as a volunteer, I experienced many events that made me realise the gaps in relation to women and development. I used to think being born as a woman is a problem in this world. I could not understand discrimination against women and young girls; it was completely unjustifiable to me, but it was like a routine matter in my culture. Most of the women would tell me, after sharing their issues and problems, that being women, it is our fate – that's why we have to bear violence and discrimination, as this has been happening to our mothers and will happen to our daughters too. I was not ready to accept this. It was not acceptable to me from any perspective.

One day, I accompanied my father to Peshawar, the capital of my province, for a meeting. Peshawar felt like a completely different place for me, even though it was a mere four hours' drive from my hometown. I saw women and young girls speaking in Urdu with confidence. I found it difficult to speak in Urdu at the time, and I couldn't imagine standing among these women with that level of confidence. When I got back to Dir, I was not at peace. I kept thinking about this gap. Why were the women and girls in my hometown struggling for their basic rights, while not so far away in Peshawar, women were seemingly free to live their lives?

Observing my surroundings more deeply, I realised that a major factor is the lack of women's representation in the decision-making process, both in the family and in society. After recognising this vacuum, I decided to establish an organisation: one not only where women could work together to improve our situation, but that would also provide a platform to represent women's issues and needs. My father and his colleagues supported me in my decision, and we established the first woman-led non-governmental organisation, Anjuman Behbood Khwateen Talash (ABKT), a women's welfare organisation. Later on, we changed the name to the Association for Behaviour and Knowledge Transformation (ABKT).

From the platform of ABKT we are striving for women's social, economic and political empowerment. We have started from a small village and now have extended our outreach to the provincial level. We have been able to engage thousands of women and girls in health, education, income generation and political empowerment-related interventions. We never forget to engage men as well, as we are aware of the fact that men are currently the decision-makers, and by ignoring them we cannot access women. Presently, ABKT is a well-recognised organisation both at national and international level for its women's empowerment efforts in the northwest of Pakistan.

What does it mean to be a Pashtun woman?

I belong to an ethnic Pashtun community inhabiting the region between the rivers Oxus in Afghanistan and Indus in Pakistan. It is known to the rest of the world through different names – Afghans, Pathans, Rohilas, and more – but the community prefers to call itself Pashtuns, or Pakhtuns.

In recent years, the world has come to know about Pakhtuns through the oppressive rule of the Taliban in Afghanistan, and especially their attitudes towards women.

Distributed over the inhospitable and harsh regions of Afghanistan and Pakistan, the Pakhtun community is perhaps the largest tribal and patriarchal society in the world today. The total population is estimated at around 40 million people, significant numbers of them in Afghanistan, Pakistan and Iran, and the rest of the world. This inward-looking society has its own folklore and, over centuries, has developed a unique unwritten social code of honour, which they call *Pakhtunwali*. *Pakhtunwali* is a subjective experience of one's own worth and an understanding of the roles and responsibilities towards each other in a tightly knit community.

Scholars have tried to define *Pakhtunwali* as consisting of three primary institutions – hospitality, *Jirga* (council of elders) and seclusion of women (*Pardah*) – however, there is no standard definition of *Pakhtunwali* with which all Pakhtuns agree. In addition to Islam, *Pakhtunwali* is the driving force that shapes individual behaviour and thoughts in Pakhtun society. It is interesting to see the interplay of Islam and *Pakhtunwali*, especially with regard to the enforcement of women's rights. The concept of *nung* or honour in *Pakhtunwali* is invariably linked to segregation and the chastity of women. The rights given to women in Islam are, for example, violated in the name of *Pakhtunwali*. As soon as a man becomes a widower, even women of the family start whispering to arrange another marriage for the widower. On the contrary, if a woman is widowed, she has two choices: either marry one of the brothers of the deceased or spend the rest of her life in *kwandtoon* or widowhood. This is against the teachings of Islam and the *Sunnah* of the Prophet of Islam. The Prophet Muhammad (PBUH) had his first marriage with a widow, Hazrat Khadija. This is one example of the inconsistencies between Islam and *Pakhtunwali*.

Women and their health

I have gathered these stories by talking to women in my region about their lives. I hoped to gain some insight into what they knew and had experienced of menopause and the place of women's health. This was my first experience of talking to women in my region about how they perceive men-opause. My conversations with them made me feel the importance of this subject, as most of these women's experiences had been difficult.

Bakhat Meena: 'It was difficult to speak with the male doctor'

I got married when I was very young. I am blessed with four sons and three daughters. My husband died in a road accident. His sudden death destroyed everything around us. I was an illiterate woman, having no source of income, nor any assets or any property that I could sell to have some money to afford basic necessities of life. That's why I started to work in agricultural fields to earn a living for my kids. My eldest son used to do labour in the market and tried to help me in providing education to his younger brothers and sisters.

Time passed, my sons and daughters got married. We lived in the same house as a big, joint family. Most of the time, when I fell ill, I didn't ask my sons to take me to the doctor for two reasons: firstly, we did not have enough money to go to the doctor, and secondly, how could I tell my son about anything related to my body and health? So, I always ignored myself.

However, when I was getting to around 45, I started getting feelings of suffocation at night. On cold winter nights, I would get wet in my sweat. I would feel like my heart was burning and beating very fast. At that time my daughters-in-law and my sons would come and try to console me by giving me water and some tablets. However, when it started becoming a daily matter, my sons got worried. That's why my eldest son, along with his wife, took me to the doctor. We didn't have female doctors, so it was difficult to speak with the male doctor. The doctors gave me medicines and later spoke to my son about my health. The next day, my daughter-in-law told me that because I was getting older, my menstruation cycle was ending and that was the reason why I had to face these symptoms. I felt very shy about what my son would think about me.

Now I am about 55 years old and I think that every woman should have information about her body and health, as most of the women in my vil-lage do not have information, because we feel shy to talk about it. We feel shy to talk about our bodies and our health. Though I have given birth to seven children, I still can't talk about my personal health issues. This may be because I never heard my mother or sisters talking to each other about such things. Though the good thing is that I have almost lived all of my life and I am still thankful to Allah for everything.

Shaista Gull: 'We women never pay attention to our health'

I got married when I was 15. I knew nothing about married life. Today, I am 29 years old. I have four kids and I don't know how I took care of myself in this entire time. All of my children were born at home with the help of a local midwife. We don't have a lady doctor in our area and my husband couldn't take me to the private hospitals because we didn't have enough money. For months I was sick after giving birth to my first girl child; her delivery was horrible. Most of the elderly women in our house would always give an example of their good health and would say, 'We never went to any doctor in our lives and gave birth to children at home, not bothering the men in the family, so why are you asking to go to the doctor?'

At the time of my marriage, I was in school. After my marriage, I couldn't continue my studies. I like to read but I can't because my life is so busy. I need to take care of eleven family members that include my children, husband and in-laws. I don't know what menopause is and have never heard about it.

♀

(I shared with Shaista Gull what menopause is and why we women need to be aware of it.)

I used to routinely go to the health awareness sessions by a local welfare organisation, where I listened to the lady health workers, who talk about women's health. But I have never heard about this before. Now, I will ask them about this when I go to that session next time. I knew that I will stop menstruating one day, but I never knew that there would be some effects of that, as you shared, and that I must also know them. Now I realise that my mother was complaining about the same symptoms, but she was not aware of why all of that was happening to her. Even today I don't know anything about menopause. We women never pay attention to our health and don't consider it important, and that is one reason why we always suffer from critical health problems, but still can't share that with anyone or talk about it.

I feel like talking about our bodies and reproductive health issues is a big sin in our culture. I don't want my daughters to experience the same things in their life. That is the reason why I am not compromising on their education and always talk to them about their health issues. My daughters are my close friends. I never had such friends when I was in my teenage years. Things have also changed quite a lot. In our house we have internet. My daughters have a laptop and they look for information and knowledge on the internet whenever they want. In our time, we didn't even have a newspaper in our house. There was a black-and-white TV, but women were not allowed to watch it. Mostly men and boys would watch TV.

Today we watch TV along with our daughters and I am happy that things are changing, and I hope my daughters will not face the problems I faced in my earlier life. They are very confident and talk to me about their problems and issues openly. I will tell my girls to learn about what menopause is and to tell me how to take care of my health when I experience it.

Fatima Jan: 'My mother thought she had a heart issue'

I got married when I was 25 years old. My husband and I are schoolteachers. After marriage, I continued my education while taking care of my children and in-laws. We are living a happy life and this is maybe because of our good financial condition. My husband is very co-operative, but this is not common in the area where I live. I support my parents financially because I don't have any brothers. I am living a good life but most of the women who are not educated and not earning themselves are not living a good life. In our area, most of the women are completely dependent on others.

Our society is very much male-dominated. Women are still struggling to create their space, that's why most women rely on men's support. What I have observed is that most of the time men do not support women. Even if they are family, they will not necessarily listen to them and provide the care they need. The example of the lives of two of my sisters is in front of me. My parents were unable to send them to school and married them off when they were very young. I am the youngest and the only daughter who was lucky enough to get schooling. But the luckiest thing was that I was able to continue my studies even after getting married. Most of the girls in my village were not given permission to continue their studies. I can take care of my needs because I have a good salary. For all my health problems I go to

Swat, a neighbouring district, to visit a lady doctor. She has been my doctor since I got married.

I came to know about menopause when my mother wasn't feeling well. She was complaining that she might have some heart issue as her heart was aching and beating fast. She was unable to sleep for many nights. I took her to my doctor. She enquired and then told me that my mother was going through menopause, which is why she was facing all these health issues. I tried to understand what menopause is and how to take care of my mother. My mother is fine now. She is quite old but still an energetic and lively lady. Whenever my mother would express her love for me, she would say, 'You are my son'. I would say that, 'No, I am your daughter and will always be your daughter.' It is not necessary to be a son to take care of your parents, rather it is to be educated, independent and caring.

I am happy that I am raising three amazing girls and two sons. I want them to become independent and also help others around them. I know how difficult it is in my culture for a woman to live a life depending on others all the time for all her needs. Most of the women in our culture are raised in a way that they are told they are not important. That is why most of the women do not consider their own health to be as important as their family's. If a woman faced any problem, she would hide it and not tell others that she needs care and support, because she believes she is not important.

Menopause: Where there are no words

Most of the women I talked to were not aware of the term 'menopause'; neither did they have any information or knowledge about it. Women had not been guided by their mothers, because their mothers were also not aware of what menopause is. They must have experienced it, but the idea of teaching your daughters or sisters about such processes is uncommon.

The overall attitude towards women's health reflects how women's issues are viewed in our society as less important than men's and are often compromised. The alarming aspect of all this is that women themselves also think that issues related to their health and bodies are not important, and that's why they do not learn about them or ask for information. Most women think that all the problems they face are their fate – and so, they don't resist. It seems as if they think about themselves as a problem. This is very disappointing. To me, the challenge is to make these women understand that their health is important to take care of and that doing so is not selfish.

Taboo conversations

I have been working with women at the grassroots level for the last twenty-four years, and still it is very difficult to engage women in these kinds of conversations, as they are raised not to talk about their bodies and health. Since their teenage years, most girls have been told to walk in a certain way, so people cannot see that they are becoming adults. That is why girls feel it is shameful to grow up. I totally understand how this affects mental and physical health. When I was growing up, my mother would also tell me not to jump, and this and that – because you are a girl, not a boy. There are many young girls who experience menstruation as their most painful life event, due to the fact that nobody tells them what menstruation is, why it happens and how they should take care of themselves while menstruating.

I myself remember when I had my first period. I was extremely upset, knowing nothing about what was happening to me. I was shivering from fear and pain for the whole day in school. I didn't move for hours, as my clothes were stained. When I came home, I rushed to talk to my friend, who lived just by my house. She told me what it all was and why it happens. She guided me to use old cloths. She also strictly said not to talk to anyone about it. I felt so bad about myself that first time, as I was clueless. This is the story of almost every growing girl.

Many women and girls carry the same experience and they never talk about it. They get married but still don't feel encouraged or confident enough to talk about issues related to their bodies and health. Among all of the women I conversed with about menopause, a very few were somehow aware of what it is, but not about its symptoms and steps for care and treatment while experiencing the process.

Out of curiosity, I did some research on the internet and found only a handful of menopause studies conducted by health practitioners and academics in Pakistan. But the language was technical and not understandable for a general reader. On YouTube, I found content mostly from India, in Hindi (although Hindi and Urdu are almost the same, so I was able to understand it). From Pakistan, again I found very few conversations on YouTube, and all of them were in Urdu. Illiteracy among women is still very high in our region, which is why the majority of women are not able to speak and understand Urdu. This made me feel worried that, despite all the development around us, we don't have sufficient and effective educational and informational material for women. This issue affects each and every woman and we should do something about it.

It is important to break the silence and start conversations about menopause. It affects many women's mental and physical health, and if they don't know about its symptoms and treatment, it becomes worse for them. During my discussions with women, I came to understand that most who have visited the doctor for menopause-related health issues – usually in case they are suffering from critical conditions – are not well guided. They have just been given painkillers, vitamins or supplements, and that's all. This is not a viable solution, in my opinion, unless and until women are educated about what, how and why menopause happens, and how they should take care of themselves and their bodies while experiencing it.

In the majority of our rural areas, there are not sufficient health facilities. There are only a few female doctors, running private clinics in the district capitals. Most women cannot afford to consult private doctors for ongoing issues, so they often prefer to visit male doctors or dispensers in their own or nearby villages, mostly in government health facilities.

I have also just recently started learning about this important matter myself, and have never really thought about it before. Now I know more about its symptoms, I have started recalling many elder women in my family and in my community who must have been experiencing the effects of menopause. But I know that most of them were unaware of this process, having no knowledge about what it is and how they can go through it with fewer effects on their mental and physical health. To my understanding, they may know about it from their own perspective, but have never heard anyone talking about it, nor can they express their feelings to others.

There is a dire need to raise awareness about this issue. Women's voices need to be heard both inside and outside their own communities, so that their bodies and the natural changes that happen to them stop being a mystery to be suffered in silence and fear.

Notes to the chapter

Information in the section 'What does it mean to be a Pashtun woman?' is taken from the book that Shad Begum is drafting about her struggle, entitled *The Circle of Fire* and due to be published during 2020.

The names of interviewees have been changed to protect their identities.

Deeply influenced by the social inequalities around her and inspired by her father's social work, **Shad Begum** has become nationally and internationally known for her determined struggle to improve the conditions of marginalised segments, especially women, of her community in north-west Pakistan. Shad is the founder and executive director of the non-profit Association for Behaviour and Knowledge Transformation (ABKT), an organisation working towards the economic and political empowerment of communities in underserved areas of Pakistan. She has worked with the UN Human Settlements Programme and UN Development Programme and, to encourage women at grassroots level, contested local elections in 2001, serving as a councillor for five years. Shad is an Ashoka Fellow, Reagan-Fascell Democracy Fellow at the National Endowment for Democracy and an Acumen Fellow. She has received numerous awards, including the US Department of State's International Women of Courage Award and the Women's World Summit Foundation Prize for Women's Creativity in Rural Life. Shad is a TED speaker and gave her first official TED talk in 2018.

7

In This Together

Sophie Watkins, menopause blogger and co-host of 'The Good, the Bad and the Downright Sweaty' podcast, and her fiancé Stephen Purvis talk with moving honesty about how Sophie's surgical menopause, due to endometriosis and premenstrual dysphoric disorder (PMDD), affected them and their lives.

Sophie

It came as no surprise to me when my consultant suggested a hysterectomy and oophorectomy (to also remove my ovaries) in March 2017. I'd been under his care since he'd diagnosed me with endometriosis at the age of 18, and in the fourteen years that followed I had endured nine laparoscopies, emergency surgery for a ruptured cyst and a caesarean section. Due to the endometriosis, I'd been given injections to induce medical menopause three times, each time offering a few months' respite from the heavy bleeding and crippling pain, but sadly the endometriosis kept returning. In 2016, my consultant diagnosed me with premenstrual dysphoric disorder (PMDD), a cyclical mood-based hormone disorder. I was experiencing a severe reaction to the natural rise and fall of oestrogen and progesterone, resulting in a week each month when my mood would rapidly change, I'd suddenly feel dangerously low, very fatigued and detached from those around me.

My own body was putting me through hell, month in, month out, and I felt so exhausted. I was so focused on a life free of endometriosis and PMDD that I didn't feel too worried about the menopause that would result from the surgery. After all, I'd been told that I'd only experience the odd hot flush or two, along with possible vaginal dryness later on in life. Little did I know ...

The intensity of the menopause symptoms that engulfed me within a day of my hysterectomy and oophorectomy still shocks me now. I recall feeling as though I was in a tropical storm: the hot flushes causing sweat to relent-lessly drip off my face and body, the racing heart making me feel afraid and as though something terrible was going to happen. I guess, in some ways, it already had. There I sat, in my hospital bed, thinking, 'What on earth have I done?' In that moment I was yet to experience being endometriosis and PMDD free; all I could think about was that I was 32 years old and had lost all of the reproductive organs I'd been born with. Even now that moment of real-isation brings tears to my eyes. I remember questioning whether I was even a woman any more, my mind tormenting me with the cruellest of questions.

To 'prepare' me for surgery I'd been in medical menopause for three years, induced with three-monthly injections of a gonadotropin-releasing hor-mone (known as GnRH; it basically switches off your ovaries). Throughout this time, I was prescribed one pump of transdermal HRT gel and had been told that this would continue after surgery. I'd been assured that the injec-tions would give me an accurate indication of how I'd feel afterwards. For me, however, this wasn't the case at all. I felt completely and utterly blind-sided and incredibly ill prepared.

The weeks that followed my surgery were a rude awakening. The tidal wave of hot flushes throughout the day were followed by unrelenting night sweats. I was generating so much heat that I joked about contacting the National Grid! Spending eighteen hours out of twenty-four soaked through was both mentally and physically draining. My partner Stephen had to buy more nighties and towels, as we couldn't keep up with the constant wash-ing and drying. Exhausted, I was left feeling utterly helpless and incredibly alone, as I didn't want to burden my friends – most of whom were either busy at home with young families or pregnant. Battling the brain fog, each day felt like Groundhog Day. Suffocated by the grogginess, my thoughts were so jumbled up that I began to struggle with straightforward tasks. I found butter in the dishwasher and the knife in the fridge. I'd go to empty the washing machine to discover I'd not actually put the washing in. On one occasion I walked to my parking space and discovered I didn't have my car keys: they were in the house, which I was now locked out of.

Prior to the surgery I was a high-functioning woman with a super-ability to multitask and recall details from a conversation I had over two weeks ago. As each day passed, I became riddled with self-doubt. I'd lost myself. One afternoon I googled 'early onset Alzheimer's', absolutely convinced that was the cause of the brain fog. Overcome with worry, I decided to book an appointment with my GP. After explaining that I was experiencing memory problems and extreme fatigue due to the night sweats, I was pre-scribed anti-depressants and sleeping tablets. All the sleeping tablets did was make me lightheaded and drowsy when I was changing the towels and my nightdress several times a night. The anti-depressants, once the initial nausea passed, did begin to help with the anxiety, so I persisted with them and I still take them now. However, they didn't address the hot flushes, night sweats, brain fog and memory loss.

Surgical menopause hugely impacted my relationships both at home and in the workplace. Being the mother of two teenage daughters, I quickly discovered that menopause and puberty don't mix. As a parent you spend the entire time praying that you're doing the right thing, hoping that your children are happy, healthy and balanced. The three of us were experienc-ing similar symptoms – irritability, mood swings and tearfulness – which most certainly caused a few clashes. Our emotions were all over the place. I experienced major mum guilt, as one moment I'd be laughing and the next, struggling to hold it all together. Before I went in for the surgery, we'd planned childcare, school runs and lifts to clubs, but I just felt so guilty as our routine went out of the window. Trying to support the girls with home-work when I couldn't remember the day of the week proved difficult. More than once I mixed up the dates of school events, resulting in many eyerolls! Mealtimes had turned into Russian roulette, as you'd never quite know what you'd end up with ... I'd either forget to add an ingredient or I'd add it twice. On one occasion I attempted to roast a chicken in a cold oven; forty-five minutes passed before I noticed. It dawned on me that while the girls knew why I'd had the surgery, they, like me, probably hadn't been expecting things to be quite so tough afterwards. So I sat them down and explained what was going on, with the help of some British Menopause Society factsheets. You always want to protect your children from the hard stuff, but they are so incredibly perceptive. After explaining why I was struggling one of my daughters said: 'Mum, you always tell us to come to you if we're sad or need help, so why haven't you come to us sooner?' I cried like a baby and learned to ask for help more, whether that was verifying what on earth I was chucking into the saucepan when I was cooking, or lugging the laundry basket around. Being honest and open helped regain balance in the house, as well as teaching both the girls and me that it's OK to ask for help.

Stephen and I were feeling the strain too. We met in April 2017 and my operation was in February 2018, so the honeymoon stage of our relationship came to an abrupt end. Stephen was nothing short of fantastic in the weeks that followed my surgery. His unwavering support made a huge difference; but again I felt overwhelmed with guilt. Having always been fiercely independent, I'd become so dependent on Stephen and, in truth, I hated it. As the weeks passed my irritability grew, along with Stephen's. He was getting very little sleep due to my constant nightie and sheet changes, and yet he still had to get up for work each day. Trying so hard to keep everything ticking over while I crumbled beside him left Stephen little time to look after his own well-being.

Despite the strain, Stephen and I ensured we kept communicating. Admittedly this sometimes led to bickering and arguments; on one occasion we argued for over half an hour ... about a light bulb. One thing I noticed quite early on in my menopause journey was how every household dispute between the four of us started to be blamed on me and my menopause, and in spite of my self-doubt I knew this was not OK. Perhaps I was the catalyst for this change, as I'd developed the unhealthy habit of apologising for everything, even if it wasn't my fault. A family meeting was called so I could raise this and – after an albeit comedic period when I became over-assertive and charged around making what I considered profound feminist statements – I calmed down and harmony was restored.

Intimacy became intermittent, due to vaginal atrophy, which I've experienced since surgery, along with a loss of libido. My libido has since been reignited, thanks to the addition of testosterone to my HRT regime. The testosterone implant, which is inserted every six months alongside my oestrogen implant, has greatly improved my cognitive function, energy levels and libido (it's also encouraged hair growth in all the wrong places – I resemble a yeti! – but thankfully the pros definitely outweigh the cons). Unfortunately, the pain and discomfort is still there, but I've recently started using a topical HRT cream, which I hope will improve things. Stephen is so supportive. There is so much emphasis on penetrative sex in the media, but intimacy is so much more than that and we've managed to stay close, even if it's just skin-to-skin contact.

Friendships began to suffer, too. I withdrew, constantly turning down invites as I didn't want anyone to see me in such a state. None of my friendship group were experiencing what I was, and I couldn't find the words to explain how I was feeling. Comments that were meant to offer reassurances unintentionally made me feel worse. Quite often I'd be told about a relative who said how 'hysterectomy was the making of her' – frustrating, as said relatives were not only twenty years older, they'd also not had their ovaries removed. On one occasion, I was asked if I was worried whether Stephen would leave me because I couldn't give him children. This hadn't crossed my mind, but planted a seed of doubt that left me feeling distraught and as though I'd failed him. When I did decide to go out for a coffee, within an hour my hair would be damp with sweat and my make-up would be sliding off my face. Everywhere felt too noisy and I became really conscious of having hot flushes in public; I'd feel as though I had a million eyes on me. Thankfully, prior to surgery I'd joined a Facebook group for women with PMDD. On this I met Cheryl, and it turned out that our surgery dates were within a week of each another. We quickly became firm friends. Cheryl was having an equally tough time adjusting to life in surgical menopause. We spoke most days and, despite being supported by my family, it was a relief to have a friend who just 'got it'.

The area of my life most affected by menopause is work. My GP gave me the all-clear to return to work six weeks post-op. Within days of my return the fatigue became overwhelming and only intensified the brain fog. This made getting through the day incredibly difficult. Every time I opened the security doors at work I could feel the stitches in my stomach pulling. At the end of each day my stomach would be so painfully swollen the commute home was torture. I recall chairing a meeting and my mind just went blank. There I stood, looking at a sea of faces, with sweat dripping down my back and upper lip, unable to recall why I was there or what the meeting was about. Thankfully a conscientious team member stepped in – I was grateful and mortified in equal parts. I felt as though I was losing my integrity and respect in the workplace. It became clear that six to eight weeks (as recommended on the NHS website) to physically recover from major abdominal surgery and removal of ovaries is by no means long enough. Setting this time frame leads to undue pressure and expectations.

I tried to return to work three more times during 2018, but each time the fatigue, exhaustion and brain fog got the better of me. It was suggested that I take an unpaid extended leave of absence; I was feeling so terrible I felt I didn't have a choice. During this time, I approached HR and asked to change my job role to one with less hours and responsibility. I struggled knowing that many of the team had seen me at my most vulnerable. HR agreed but I still had to apply for the new role and go through the company's stringent interview process, which involved three notoriously difficult aptitude tests. To my utter relief and surprise, I passed all three and was offered the alternative role. It was the best decision I could have made. The lower income has taken a while to adjust to, but my work–life balance has improved and I feel so much happier. In January 2019, I returned to work and the new team is fantastic. I am one of two women in a team of twenty-one. I've educated them (at length) about menopause, as everyone will know someone who is experiencing it and understanding needs to be improved, especially in the workplace. They're all incredibly supportive and have become dab hands at saying, 'Yes Sophie, it's boiling hot in here', when I exclaim about how warm it is. Even though I can see them sat there in coats, it makes me feel better!

One of the biggest frustrations of surgical menopause is the difficulty in accessing menopause support. It seems to be a postcode lottery. Unfortunately, after my surgery there was no post-op follow-up appointment and I was discharged back to the care of my GP. As GP menopause training isn't mandatory, my GP didn't feel equipped to make decisions about changing my HRT, so referred me back to the gynaecologist who did my surgery. But I was told it could take months. I broke down in the surgery. I felt so utterly helpless. The next day the mental health crisis team was sent to our house. I felt afraid and fearful: what if they admitted me into hospital? Refusing to let them into the house, I stood on our cottage doorstep in my porridge-smeared (and slightly stinky) pyjamas. On reflection, the poor team at the door were great; they listened and actually weren't surprised I felt so awful. Leaving me with a card, they told me to ring if I felt any worse. It left me wondering how many other women have been unnecessarily referred to mental health services when they in fact need to be seen by a menopause specialist.

I recognised that I could do with talking things through, but a search for a local menopause support group returned no results. A chance visit to my local haberdashery led to the beginning of The Menopause Club. While having a good old natter with the lovely shopkeeper, Kim, I had the biggest hot flush. As I stripped off (not literally), Kim said: 'I know exactly how you feel'. I touched on how much I was struggling and mentioned that I wanted to start a club. Kim offered me the use of her workshop, one evening a month. Open to anyone, we invited people to join us to chat about menopause while doing a craft activity. We made posters and asked to advertise in local GP surgeries and pharmacies. Bizarrely a few refused, as we weren't an 'NHS-led group'. I found that incredibly disappointing. Surely such groups could actually reduce the pressure on the NHS?

Looking back, I'm surprised I was able to begin a group when I felt so desperate, but it made a huge difference being able to talk with people who just understood. I'm not a health professional and always make that clear, but what the group offers is a safe space to speak freely about menopause. We signpost to the NICE guidelines, British Menopause Society and Menopause Support. Women shouldn't have to fight so hard to receive adequate help and support. I spent my days off reading menopause advice and literature, but others may feel overwhelmed by the information that's available, some of which can be contradictory and confusing. Understanding of menopause in the UK is definitely changing for the better: GPs are choosing to undertake training, media coverage has grown, taboos are being broken down and companies are beginning to introduce menopause in the workplace guidelines.

A plea for help on social media led to the beginning of feeling better for me. I posted a tweet that was answered by the lovely Diane Danzebrink. Diane and I spoke on the phone, and that call was the start of feeling like 'me' again. After my requests to be referred to an NHS menopause clinic were refused, I decided to go further into my overdraft and visited a private doctor. It felt great to be understood, and blood tests showed that my oestrogen level was non-existent – the low level of HRT I was taking wasn't enough. Discovering that I wasn't losing my mind filled me with relief and hope. It transpired that my body was absorbing the HRT erratically, sending me on an emotional rollercoaster – and I've never been a fan of rides! When attempts at raising my oestrogen levels through conventional HRT failed, Dr Hannah Short requested that my GP refer me for a HRT implant. They initially made me feel as though I was pregnant – a cruel reminder of what I could no longer have – but after two weeks I could feel myself lifting. The night sweats stopped, the hot flushes began to subside and, most of all, I had mental clarity. Every six months I head to the menopause clinic and have my implant replaced. I always get a hormone dip before their renewal, which takes me straight back to those weeks immediately after my surgery, but they offer me stability and have improved my well-being considerably.

As you've read, adapting to life with surgical menopause has been a challenge. While I don't think anything could have fully prepared me for how I'd feel after surgery, I definitely think more needs to be done to give women factual, up-to-date, evidence-based information prior to life-changing surgery. A hot flush or two just doesn't even begin to touch on the menopause symptoms I've experienced. It's common for women in surgical menopause to suffer the extremities of menopause and I just wish that I'd been given the opportunity to prepare myself mentally for the challenges ahead. While it is great to be endometriosis and PMDD free, I didn't realise until after surgery that my endometriosis could come back. Nor did I know that for women with a history of PMDD, regaining hormone balance in menopause can be a rollercoaster.

In spite of my struggles, there is a silver lining, the joy of new friendships and the opportunity to take a step back and evaluate my life. Over the past two years I've met so many incredible women. The Menopause Club in Hitchin became so popular that I've since started a second group and have further planned throughout the UK. I think it's beautiful how a group of complete strangers bonded over menopause; we've all seen one another at our most vulnerable and have cried, laughed and grown together. If it wasn't for menopause, I wouldn't have met the lovely Diane, Cheryl, Kim and Kayleigh who I now consider dear friends.

If you're struggling, my biggest piece of advice is don't give up! Arm yourself with knowledge, self-advocate and reach out and talk about it; you're not alone. Join a Facebook group, attend a Menopause Café or a Menopause Club – the power of being able to speak freely with people who just 'get it' is huge. Alongside this I've also learned about self-care. Up until recently I've always struggled to say no, so worried that I would disappoint or upset people, I neglected to put my own needs and well-being first. It's been empowering to discover that it's OK to say no. Years ago I'd love nothing more than a night out with dancing and cocktails, whereas now I much prefer a quiet meal out or a trip to the cinema. It's given me the opportunity to achieve a better work–life balance and despite causing temporary strain in my relationships, it has actually brought us all closer. Stephen proposed at the end of 2018; after asking him whether he was sure I said a big 'YES' and we're planning our wedding for 2021. We're beyond excited.

Menopause prompted me to make healthier lifestyle choices earlier on than I perhaps would have. My body thinks it's 50 so I learned that I have to 'nourish to flourish'. Most of all I've learned how to be kind to myself. I think many women are guilty of putting their own happiness last, focusing on pleasing everyone else instead. That's changed for the better, and about time too!

Stephen

Sophie and I met more than three years ago now, on an online dating site. Chatting online, we hit it off immediately. After speaking on the phone, we planned our first date. We went for a romantic meal in a restaurant that is now one of our favourite 'date night' locations. Both of us were visibly nervous; my hands wouldn't stop shaking.

It was during our third date that Sophie asked me whether I wanted to have children in the future and my answer was, 'If children happen, then great ... but I'm at that age in my life where I'm approaching 40, and I never wanted to be an old dad.' I couldn't see myself running around at 50 with bad knees trying to play football and keep up with a young child; instead I gained incredible twin stepdaughters, who I love dearly. Hearing my response, Sophie then broached the subject of being in induced menopause through medication which was preparing her for surgery. Although it was worrying, my mum had an early hysterectomy and it wasn't going to put me off. As we grew closer, we had open and honest conversations about what was to come. Recognising it would be a challenging and tough time for Sophie, I had no doubt in my mind that I wanted to support her every step of the way.

Sophie's surgery was first scheduled for August 2017. I remember her being really, really anxious. In the period running up to the surgery I had noticed the deterioration in her health. When we first met, she was really into walking and was training to do a marathon distance charity mountain walk. But in the months getting closer to surgery she was struggling to walk and would often pass out. On one occasion she knocked herself out and the girls had to call me to come over and help. Sophie was experiencing a lot of pelvic and abdominal pain. There was a clear need for the surgery because it was having a direct impact on her quality of life. Initially, she was having the GnRH injections that induced menopause every four weeks, but this changed to every three weeks as the injections kept wearing off, and she would begin bleeding and become agitated, withdrawn and very anxious.

As Sophie was having an abdominal hysterectomy, we started making plans for after the surgery. At the time I lived in a two-bedroom flat in Hitchin, where everything was on one floor, as opposed to Sophie's charming, yet impractical cottage with uneven floors and low ceilings that I constantly hit my head on. The original plan was that Sophie would move in with me for six weeks, as it would be easier for her to get to the toilet, in and out of bed, have baths and showers, and the girls could come over and visit and stay at weekends. All of our plans proved fruitless, however, as the operation was cancelled, leaving Sophie distraught. She was angry, saying things like, 'I just want the pain, bleeding and emotional instability to stop. I don't know how much more I can take.' She was really worried about work as they'd employed a contractor to cover her leave. In spite of this, we continued making plans; we found a beautiful little two-and-a-half-bedroom house and moved in together. It was great – stressful, obviously, with the worry about what was going to happen with the surgery – but the house gave us what we needed and also meant the girls could stay at home while Sophie recovered from surgery.

At the time, I worked away three days a week. When the new surgery date came through, I organised to work from home for the next four or five weeks, only to have the surgery cancelled again. Sophie fell to pieces and felt extremely guilty, as she could see me getting stressed with work.

Eventually, on the day the surgery finally went ahead, I remember waking up feeling terrified, given that past operations hadn't been straightforward for Sophie. There'd been problems with haemorrhaging when she had a caesarean and her tonsils removed, so I was understandably anxious, but at the same time I had to be supportive and try not to show that fear. That morning, we heard tickets were going on sale for Lionel Ritchie, so I bought tickets for Brighton – literally just as we were leaving the house – to give Sophie something to look forward to. At the hospital, I took her up for her check-in. Soon after our arrival, someone came in and said, 'Sophie, could you come to this room ...' and at that point I wasn't allowed to go through. Sophie messaged me to say she was going in for the surgery, but that was the last I heard about how she was doing for about eight hours.

Feeling worried and nervous, I recall constantly checking my phone. We'd been told she'd be in surgery for an hour or two, and that she should be on the ward around half-past three or four o'clock, but it was quarter to seven before I received a call telling me Sophie was in recovery. As soon as I received the call I rushed over to the hospital. I arrived as she was wheeled on to the ward and felt so happy – and relieved to see her. I told her 'I love you,' and despite Sophie's drug-induced grogginess, she said she loved me too.

We were told the recovery period for Sophie's op was usually six to eight weeks, but in reality it's six to eight weeks just for the scars to start healing. When we first arrived home, it was clear that there was very little that Sophie could do for herself. I needed to be there, to make drinks, take up breakfast in the morning, bring lunch – there was a lot to do. The hot flushes – which Sophie wasn't expecting – were endless. Sophie was exhausted as she was also struggling to sleep at night. I get pretty hot anyway, so when I went anywhere near her she would push me away, as she was too hot from the relentless night sweats.

Sophie spoke to other people who'd had their ovaries removed, and it seemed as though everyone was struggling. She started researching what people had gone through, and what a long road she could be in for, and began to deeply regret the decision she had made. She forgot all the bad things leading up to why she had the surgery – which I kept trying to remind her of – and was focusing on the negative aspects. It was a really tough period for Sophie; she felt as though she was letting both the girls and me down and shed a lot of tears. Spending so much time lost in her own thoughts, she became frustrated that she was unable to be her usual active and sociable self and would get really distressed when she'd forget words or what she was talking about mid-sentence.

It's difficult when you can see that your partner is in pain and emotionally struggling, yet you're unable to console them or offer the reassurances they need, because I too felt so ill prepared for the sheer magnitude of symptoms Sophie was experiencing and I sometimes just couldn't find the right words. All I could do was hug Sophie, or hold her hand if she was too hot to be held. Sophie kept apologising, and I would say: 'There's no need to apologise, you've done nothing wrong.'

At one point I was so wiped out, I felt absolutely exhausted. I would frequently fall asleep while watching TV downstairs. There is an expectation that men just keep and calm and carry on. No one asked me how I was, but seeing the woman I love struggle through every minute of a day crushed me. I felt floored by it, made worse by my own tiredness and the growing list of things to do on top of my day job. I remember one of Sophie's friends coming round and saying, 'OK, I'm going to make cups of tea. Do you want a drink, Stephen?' I really appreciated it, as it momentarily took the pressure off me and gave me a little bit of respite.

The first time we were intimate again, we were both excited, and nervous, given experiences we'd had in the past, as intercourse had become quite painful due to Sophie's endometriosis. We weren't sure how it was going to go, but, to our surprise – and enjoyment – it went really well. Sophie often asked me, 'Does it feel any different than before?' She was worried about dryness, because she had heard that can happen after surgery, but that wasn't a problem at that time.

Just as things started to settle, it was time for Sophie to return to work and life quickly became unsettled again as it became apparent that eight weeks' recovery just wasn't enough. Work was a real struggle, especially with being in such a stressful environment where people expect you to be on the ball straight away. She would come home incredibly upset and say she just didn't know how to do her job any more, and I would try to reassure her that wasn't the case: 'You're really intelligent and so capable, you just need to give it time.'

During a planned trip to Italy, travelling from Venice on to Florence and Rome, it became clear that the journey ahead was going to be much tougher than we anticipated. Sophie was tearful, exhausted from the lack of sleep and she was still in so much discomfort and her stomach was painfully swollen. She feared she was holding us back on that holiday, but we had to keep reassuring her that, actually, you're not: this is a holiday for all of us together, and there'll be certain things that we can or can't do.

I think the most stressful thing I found was dealing with doctors, the NHS and trying to get Sophie the right help. The one thing I would recommend, if someone is approaching this or their partner will be going through a hysterectomy, is to ensure that you ask for the care beforehand and try to make sure that you've got the right level of hormone treatment, so all that is planned up front – because for Sophie, there was no post-care. The other thing I would recommend is that although they say six to eight weeks for recovery, plan for being off work longer than that, for some it's as much as six to nine months, and in hindsight, it's something we should have budgeted for.

After our trip to Italy in May, we were left feeling anxious about a California road trip we had planned for September. Just before going, we had some good news: Sophie had been referred to the Chelsea and Westminster Menopause Clinic. The road trip was fantastic, especially as one afternoon in a vineyard, I got down on one knee and proposed. Sophie kept saying, 'Are you sure?' and I replied, 'I love you more than ever'. Prior to proposing I'd asked the girls' permission and, after agreeing, they practised proposing with the ring, much to my bemusement! As a family we'd been through a challenging period, yet through it all we'd managed to stay close, joke, laugh and have fun together.

For those with young families, I would say prioritise what's important, and plan easy, quick meals, so you're not having to spend two hours preparing food. If you can take time off work, and not have to worry about those stresses, that can help support your partner at home. Especially in the first few weeks, I was having to help out a lot with changing dressings and providing childcare cover and the endless washing. It also means you'll be more able to help them if they're struggling with insomnia – at least then they can get up and you won't have to worry about being up at six o'clock or seven o'clock for work the next day.

Not long after we got back from the US, Sophie's pain intensified and she was complaining of general bone ache and body pain. Worried about bone density, she had a DEXA bone scan. Thankfully it was good, but she has since been diagnosed with fibromyalgia, which she is trying to manage through exercise. Sophie had repeated urine infections as well, some of which occurred after we had intercourse, so I began to worry that I was causing the pain which left her feeling uncomfortable

Prior to the vaginal atrophy issues, it had felt almost like we were going back to normality, but then that was taken away. We get anxious before having any form of intimacy. Sophie worries that she is letting me down, that's she done something wrong and thinks I'll leave her if she can't satisfy me, which isn't true. I know she's beautiful, I know she's amazing, and I just don't ever want to do things that are going to hurt her. So, because I've associated sex with putting Sophie through pain, I think it's been quite hard for us to remain intimate at times. Sometimes when I've held back, Sophie has said she felt it was me rejecting her, whereas in fact it's me not wanting to put pressure on her. In hindsight, I think we probably should have been communicating more around that topic, because it can become a vicious cycle.

Sometimes I've had to be more of the realist in the relationship. Sophie had very high hopes of a settled and pain-free life after surgery, which were then dashed. I think, as any partner, that one thing you have to keep reminding your other half of is that actually, before you had this surgery, you were really unwell. Although you may have these other challenges to contend with now, it's different to what you had in the past. Also – and the doctors have said we should stop doing this – Sophie has come to blame any illness she has on menopause. But the menopause isn't the cause of all problems in the world, and sometimes there are other things happening to your body that you need to get looked at and investigated properly. That's where partners can really come in, to say, actually, what you're going through here isn't anything to do with menopause.

For a couple where the woman is experiencing vaginal atrophy, or symptoms making intimacy impossible, or not something that they want to do, what I would recommend is to always remain close. We always enjoy spending time with one another. We're always cuddling up on the sofa and giving each other hugs. I think you've got to retain that closeness, and that closeness isn't just about sex. It's about massages, holding hands, being intimate with each other, talking to each other. It's about having fun experiences together. And if we can have sex as well sometimes, then that's great.

The other thing is that you need to look forward. It's so easy at times, when going through periods like we have in the past two years, to look back and over-analyse and over-critique, and that can bring a lot of depressive thoughts. You've always got to look to more positive times in the future. If we compare where we are now to two years ago, we'd probably both admit to each other that we're in a much better place.

What Sophie has done is amazing. She realised that there's very little support network around here. So she started her own support group, and it's turned out to be one of the best things that she could have done. The clubs have proven really popular. Sophie has been able to take her experiences and actually help others, as well as getting help from them – even though they probably don't realise it at times, they're helping her, by sharing their stories.

I never feel as if Sophie talks too much about menopause. I'll always be a listening ear. She may sometimes worry that she bores everyone with it but that definitely isn't the case. The Menopause Support forums have been a huge help to Sophie as they're so relatable and it helps to talk about it with people who just 'get it'. As much as I can try, I'll never fully know what Sophie is going through, because it's happening to her, not me. Communication is crucial, as are cuddles! I'm excited for our future and I know Sophie is too.

With a history of endometriosis and PMDD, **Sophie Watkins** is passionate about supporting women through their menopause. She is eager to share factual, evidence-based information both in the community and the workplace and is the founder of The Menopause Club Hitchin and Biggleswade. Alongside this, Sophie co-hosts 'The Good, the Bad and the Downright Sweaty' podcast. Aged 34, Sophie is mother to teenage twin daughters and fiancée to Stephen. Sophie is a lover of flowers and can usually be found pottering about in the garden when she's not at work as a business officer in a large defence company. A self-confessed craft addict, she enjoys painting and getting creative, although she admits she quite often ends up with more paint in her hair than on the canvas! Travel is Sophie's greatest joy; keen to share menopause information globally, she always takes a stack of menopause information leaflets along for the ride.

Stephen has been Sophie's partner since 2017 and is stepdad to her two teenage girls. He is an IT geek for a global firm, a keen cyclist and car enthusiast – the faster the better! Born in Whitley Bay, Stephen is also a huge Newcastle United supporter. A foodie, wine and whisky connoisseur, he enjoys travelling the world and experiencing new cultures.

8

A Time of Letting
the Baggage Go

Carren Strock describes herself as an all-round Renaissance Woman, and as a writer she is probably best known for her groundbreaking book *Married Women Who Love Women*, now in its third edition. Hers is an exploration of menopause and the love we find during midlife.

I grew up knowing that I was supposed to marry a nice man who would be a good provider and a good father. And I did just that. I'd been married for twenty-five years when I fell in love with my best friend, some years before I reached menopause. Anyway, she didn't feel the same way about me and I went on a quest to find out if it was just her I was in love with, or if I was a lesbian. I discovered the latter.

As a period is our body's way of releasing tissue that it no longer needs to prepare us for pregnancy, menopause is nature's way of releasing that excess baggage we've harboured for years, preparing us for the next part of our lives. The baggage might be almost anything: a grief we've never fully acknowledged, an unfilled desire that has been eating at us, or, as in my case, a secret knowing that I was not the person everyone believed me to be ... you fill in your own blank. Sometimes that baggage is so deeply embedded that we don't even realise we're carrying it until we begin our passage through perimenopause, the time in which our ovaries gradually begin to make less oestrogen. We begin to experience changes in period cycles. Hot flushes, sleep disturbances and mood swings become routine for some. Our skin becomes so thin, literally, and we become so highly sensitive and vulnerable, that all of the 'stuff' we've been harbouring rises to the surface and we can cry at the drop of a hat.

Most women begin this journey in their mid-forties. I think I was around 50 when my menopause arrived. I know it was after I realised that I was gay. If anyone who knew what I was going through asked how I was, I'd become an emotional wreck. The only way I could describe what was happening to me was by comparing my body to a taut balloon. It felt as though there was one tiny pin-prick in me from which all of the emotional 'stuff' was slowly oozing out. I cried more than I ever had in my entire life, but through it all I came out a stronger woman. And so, when I went through menopause, it was a breeze.

I believe that the emotional baggage that might have come out during my menopause came out earlier because of my discovery, and so my menopause was smooth sailing. But at the time I desperately needed to find a place for my feelings to be and I wrote this:

The Secret
In the space of a short time – that seemed forever,
I had become a stranger.
But so artful was I at hiding my secret that no one knew.
I'd sit in a room peopled with old friends and feel invisible.
My family talked to the woman I had been,
unaware of the woman I'd become.
I'd see myself on a darkening highway,
walking the yellow line.
If I stepped to the right,
the stoic, confident me came forth.
If I veered to the left,
toward the few who knew the truth,
my tears would flow.

When I first came out in 1988, I had no idea as to what to do. I spoke with as many gay women as I could find. Some said I had to leave my marriage.

Some said I didn't. I came to the realisation that what I had discovered about myself was simply another dimension. Telling my husband definitely put a strain on our relationship. Still, my marriage had been a good one and I didn't want to leave it. Difficult in the beginning, through much communication, we had redefined our relationship. We are still together many years later and I am an out lesbian. Recently, my daughter said to me, 'I think you and daddy have the best marriage of anyone I know, because you really talk to each other.'

When I realised that not all married women who love women leave their marriages, I began to explore the different ways in which women led their lives. That brought me to write the book I am best known for, *Married Women Who Love Women*, now in its third edition. The majority of the women I interviewed in the early 1990s were in their mid-thirties to their mid-fifties when their same-sex feelings became apparent – just about the time many were going through perimenopause or entering menopause.

The main thing I've learned about menopause is that it is consistently inconsistent. I put the word out on the numerous online groups I belong to, asking for women who wanted to share their menopause stories. Very few people shared identical experiences. The luckier ones said, 'it was easy' or, 'nothing really exceptional'. Several said, 'My period just stopped.'

We, as women, are all unique. I was at dinner one winter evening with seven friends. All of us had gone through menopause. Outdoors, the temperature was a brisk 32° Fahrenheit (0°C). Yet as I looked around the table in the restaurant, I had to laugh. One woman wore a tank top and complained that it was too hot. One kept her winter jacket on. I wore a heavy sweater. The rest were clothed somewhere in between. Other than the woman in the tank top, we were all comfortable – for the moment.

The show *Menopause the Musical* is a parody that finds the humour in a woman's 'change of life', when four ladies with little in common meet at a lingerie sale in a department store. They poke fun at their hot flushes, forgetfulness, mood swings and night sweats, and these diverse women create a sisterhood as they realise that menopause is a shared experience that doesn't have to be suffered in silence.

All of the people I have spoken with, either through my call-out or in casual conversation, could have been in that show. While it was happening, they saw nothing funny about what they were going through, but now they could laugh at the inopportune times their flushes chose to show themselves – in front of a class of junior high school students, during an important business meeting, in bed with someone special. These were the first things women said when I asked them about their menopause:

> I gave away every turtle-neck and pull-on sweater I owned. I needed to be able to open or close, zip and unzip, fast. The season in my body could change in an instant.

> I lost ten pounds in two years, just pulling my blankets on and off, on and off, all night long.

> Every time I walked into a room I'd say, 'Is it hot in here or is it me?'

> My entire body, the perspiration dripped from it. Under my breasts, and I have large breasts. I was in and out of the shower.

> Sometimes I was so hot I'd run into my car just to put the air-conditioner on. I needed immediate cold.

Dorathea's sweats were so bad that she carried a change of clothes with her when she went out – until she spent a week with friends who ate only vegan. She ate what they did, and her sweats stopped. She has since become a vegan herself. What Dorathea learned was not surprising. Hot flushes and night sweats occur before and during menopause because of changing hormone levels, including oestrogen and progesterone, which affect the body's temperature control. Certain seeds, fruits, vegetables, soy products and oils are known to boost oestrogen levels and they are found in vegan diets.

While hot flushes and nocturnal sweats are most memorable for some, others talked about chocolate cravings, lapses in memory and sexual problems. At about the same time we are experiencing our first encounters with menopause, many other things are going on in our immediate worlds. Most of us have raised our kids, are going through empty nest syndrome and beginning to think about the next part of our lives. From having no memory of going through their menopause to remembering all too well, women ran the gamut. One said, 'I remember every day. I'm 71 and still get hot flashes.' She isn't alone. Some women continue to get hot flushes years after they've passed their last period.

Many lesbians felt there was a connection between their coming out and menopause. Those who had been married wondered if there had been signs they'd just ignored while busy doing what they were supposed to be doing as wives and mothers. They wondered if they had been playing a role while raising their children. They spoke of the chaos and confusion in their lives at that time – kids leaving home, older parents needing care, retirement looming ahead. It became obvious to some that they were in stuck places and just not happy. Whether or not they thought they might be attracted to women, it was at that time in their lives that they felt an overwhelming need to make changes: return to school, leave their marriages, find more challenging jobs. One woman talked of having an epiphany when she reached menopause. She realised that her time on earth was limited and her life was passing her by. So being true to herself became her main objective.

Maria realised that she was attracted to women in college and identified as bisexual for most of her life. Her husband knew before he married her in the 1980s. She said:

We focused on our careers and raised two kids together. I suppressed my attraction to women for three decades until I decided – after thirty years of marriage, a year and a half after the hysterectomy that triggered the start of menopause, one year after becoming an empty nester, and six months after my mother's death – that I did not want to suppress my attraction to women any longer. After more than a year of therapy, I now have a girlfriend. I hope to preserve my marriage and maintain my relationship with my girlfriend forever. They have met and like each other but my relationship with each of them is separate. We are navigating our situation better than most.

Another woman reflected:

Menopause and gayness came about almost simultaneously. I thought it was menopause that was causing me to feel the way I was feeling. It also coincided with my mother falling deeper into dementia and not knowing who I was. I think that had a lot to do with me waking up to who I authentically was. I've had it in my mind, for many years, that I would start to uncouple from my husband when our daughter graduated high school. She turned 18 last week and the reality of that happening hit me harder than I thought it would.

I asked other women if they'd experienced their emotional baggage surfacing before they'd reached menopause and if they thought that had changed them. Those who were living authentic lives, who were comfortable with themselves and with their bodies, and who had supportive and loving partners (male or female) with whom they could share this 'insanity', reported having an easier time with it.

Doctors have mistakenly believed that it is natural for menopausal women who are not sexually active to lack sexual drive. Women bought into this belief that menopause brings decreased sexual functioning. But the reasons women are not sexually active are varied. It might be the discomfort brought on by dryness, which can often be easily alleviated. But it could also be that there is no available partner, or maybe it is an unsatisfying marriage – in which case, menopause is a good excuse to cease sexual activities. As one woman so aptly put it, 'I went through menopause right after I came out. The pause of mena was definitely life-changing.'

When girls begin to menstruate they learn that this is a sign they are physically capable of becoming pregnant. Likewise, some women see menopause as a sign that they are no longer a full woman: 'I knew exactly when I had my last period. It was heavier than any period I had ever had. For one split second I felt bad. I could never have another baby. I felt like I had lost the ability to feel like a real woman. I felt as though sexually I was facing an end.'

Other women have rejoiced upon reaching this point. Some heterosexual women in good relationships noted an increase in sexual activity as, no longer fearful of unwanted pregnancies, they felt freer to enjoy sex. Weight gain, which frequently happens during menopause, hampered the enjoyment for others, however, because cultural ideals equate being thin with being desirable. Some of the women who identified as lesbian or bisexual seemed to be less concerned with their body images, as they were less affected by cultural ideals of what a woman should look like. While other women found little or no correlation between their sexual desires and passing menopause, it was at this stage of their lives that they chose to leave unsatisfying marriages and find more compatible mates. And some ended up having better sex than ever before:

I remember my menopause. I had this girlfriend. We had sex the first time we were together. The sex part of our relationship was amazing. Orgasms every time – for both of us. I was having hot flashes and I was tired most of the time and my periods were on again and off again, so I figured that I was in my menopause but thank God my sexual libido stayed intact.

Deep inside I've known and had these feelings my whole life. I was teased for being a lesbian in junior high. Crushed on and later obsessed about girls, and then women until I finally broke the closet door down at 46. That said, menopause hasn't diminished (maybe enhanced?) my sex drive.

My first relationship with another woman was after I began my menopause at 55.

I think I'm in perimenopause. My periods are a bit sporadic. Otherwise no symptoms, unless becoming gay is a symptom of perimenopause.

I think hormone fluctuations caused me to be a little more randy than I normally would be.

Most women begin menopause naturally, but menopause can also come about due to a great many variables. Anything that damages your ovaries or stops oestrogen production can cause early menopause. That includes chemotherapy for cancer, the removal of ovaries, a total hysterectomy, pre-diabetic shots, or drugs. Thyroid disorders may also cause the early onset of menopause or be mistaken for early menopause. Harriet said:

I felt tired all of the time, forgetful, and I was having mood swings. I also gained weight, my menstrual cycles became irregular, and I had little tolerance for cold. When I took a blood test, they found I had an underactive thyroid, so I assumed everything I was experiencing was because of my thyroid. I had no idea that the symptoms for both thyroid dysfunction and menopause were so similar. My menopause came about because of my thyroid problem.

Jill, at 39, became moody, emotional. She began to experience a lot of anxiety, which turned into panic attacks:

I remember I became apprehensive about flying. If I drank glass of wine, I'd get a headache. My suits were getting tighter, I was gaining weight, my metabolism was slowing down. I had ovaries, but I had had my uterus removed, so it took me some time before I realised that I was going through menopause.

Felicia, a trans man, said:

I definitely noticed my menopause, because it was surgically induced. I had cancer and whatever plumbing I had left was removed. I had very mixed feelings about it. I was relieved because I never wanted those parts, and I've always had issues with them not working right in some way, physically. I had several days of agony every month for decades. Oddly, I did sort of notice my lesbianism and trans-ness around that time.

The symptoms of menopause can certainly cause stress, but stress itself can also promote early menopause. For example, women who live under economic hardship are more likely to experience early menopause: 'As soon as I left my husband, I started menopause ... at 40. Very stressful time of my life!'

♀

It would be unfair to talk about menopause without also talking about periods, because menopause is the end result of the period – that first, sometimes terrifying venture into the world of womanhood. When I asked women if they had a vivid recollection of their menopause, most were vague, because menopause didn't just happen. It continued to happen over a long time. But that first period – splat. It arrived. Menstruation, although traversed in silence, secrecy and taboos, is a passage that women never forget.

When I first got my period, I figured boys must get something too. I remember asking my mother, 'If girls get periods, what do boys get?' My mother said, 'I don't know. I'll ask your father.' She never came back to me with an answer.

In Judaism, when a boy turns 13, he goes through the Bar Mitzvah ceremony. This symbolises that he has become a man and is now responsible for his own actions. Before the Bar Mitzvah, his parents hold that responsibility. I had just turned 11 the night before my brother's Bar Mitzvah. I saw blood on my panties and called my mother. She came into the bathroom and asked me if I had done anything down there to hurt myself. I said no.

She smiled, then gave me a gentle slap. 'It's custom,' she said, to explain the slap. Although the custom is widespread, the reasons vary from: when you bleed the blood rushes from your face and your cheeks become pale, so the slap brings a flush back to your cheeks, to: by slapping a girl the blood rushes to her cheeks so less is shed below.

At the temple for my brother's Bar Mitzvah service the following morning, each time a prayer called for us to rise, I visualised the wad of cotton between my vulval lips falling to the floor and everyone knowing my secret. But what happened was even more embarrassing. My mother and I were sitting with the women in our family and I saw her mouth the words 'Carren got her period' to all of my aunts and cousins. I didn't appreciate at the time that as my brother was being welcomed into the world of men, I had taken my rite of passage into the world of women. What could be more memorable than that?

Years ago, I belonged to a consciousness-raising group. The sense of sisterhood that grew from our meetings became so strong that no topic was off limits. One evening we shared stories of our first menses. In our thirties and forties at the time, we all had vivid memories. The more we described our early experiences – figuring out how to put on sanitary belts and attach pads, or how to keep rewashed rags or wads of cotton from dropping to the floor – the more hysterical we became. By the time one woman told us about trying to insert a tampon we were howling. Panicked, she'd screamed to her mother on the other side of the door: 'I can't find my hole!'

Some first periods had comfortable memories attached to them while others made us cringe. Charlotte told us that she was raised in a convent. One morning she woke up, got out of bed and saw blood on the front of her night gown. Not knowing what to do, she got back into bed. When the nun came to wake the girls, she threw off Charlotte's covers and saw the red stain. 'You can stay in bed,' she said, replacing the covers. Charlotte, believing she was dying, remained in bed all day. It was only after classes, when the others returned to the dorm they all shared, that one of the older girls explained what was happening.

Lianna talked of living with her grandmother. Her only sex education had been the warning, 'If you let any boy touch you down there, you will bleed and get pregnant.' When Lianna saw blood on her panties she thought she was pregnant and told her grandmother, who promptly threw her out of the house.

Mandy recalled:

I must have known what was happening because I wasn't frightened when I saw the blood. I don't know why, as I think back, but at the time, I didn't tell anyone. I used tissues to stop the flow. Then I found a box of tampons my mother and older sister used and I figured out how to use them. It's funny – neither of them ever questioned that the box needed to be replaced more often.

What was remarkable was that, after that night of sharing and sisterhood, within a week, we all had our periods – even the women who believed they had entered menopause.

As human beings we continually struggle, torn between wanting to be who we really are, and wanting to be who we feel we are supposed to be. We often fake what we don't feel, and say yes when we want to say no. But once a woman discovers who she really is, or comes to terms with her same-sex sexuality, she can no longer pretend.

When I moved, I met Marge, who became an instant friend. She was always asking me to visit but, every time I did, she spent the day complaining about everything you could think of. She never had a nice word to say about anyone and each time I left her house I felt drained. Once I came to realise who I was, and accept myself, I began to experience a kind of increased self-confidence. I reached a point where I was finally able to love myself unconditionally and I began to not care so much about other people's opinions, acceptable convention and niceness. And it suddenly dawned on me: I could choose not to spend time with Marge. (Thinking about this now, years later, and knowing more about menopause, I wonder if Marge was dealing with her own perimenopausal hormone changes.) What came to me, in a sort of 'a-ha' way, was what I call my three truths:

1. No one knows what I am thinking unless I say the words.
2. I just show up. No expectations – no disappointments.
3. If someone can't deal with who or what I am, the problem is theirs, not mine. I no longer concern myself with the disparaging opinions of others.

These realisations have empowered me; they've given me a new-found freedom, and the ability to walk to the beat of my own drum. And I am no longer afraid to say whatever it is I want to say.

I was waiting for my yearly mammogram when an older woman walked into the waiting room. She told me she'd had to take a day off from work and drink a ton of water for her pelvic ultrasound. She was so nervous she'd forgotten to bring the doctor's referral letter and the receptionist, an arrogant young woman, said, 'Sorry. You have to come back'.

The old woman, head down, turned to leave. 'Wait a minute,' I said, my dander suddenly rising at the injustice of this. I jumped out of my seat. 'No one comes in off the street and asks for a pelvic ultrasound. You call her doctor. He can fax her letter.'

The receptionist dialled, then said: 'He's not in.' Again the woman turned toward the exit. 'No. Don't leave,' I said to her. Turning to the uninterested receptionist, I demanded to speak to the manager, and then to her superior. Long story short, the test was approved. The old woman, surprised, said to me, 'I didn't know I was allowed to do that.'

My heart went out to this woman. There was a time in my life when I too followed directions, even those I felt unjust. I would have been afraid to speak up for myself, let alone for a stranger. I believe that coming out, and then arriving at my menopause, and owning that real me, created that power.

Ageing and menopause used to be linked together. A woman in menopause was expected to be irritable, tired, depressed, or all three. And we fed into that ageist culture. Commercials told us that we would fall apart if we were not on some sort of medication. And we believed those, too. Pharmaceutical companies preyed on us. They still do, but fortunately, our beliefs about age have shifted dramatically in the last decade. We are now seeing more media coverage of the strong, energetic menopausal women we are. We are looking younger and sexier than ever before and we are changing our cultural negativity about ageing and menopause.

Notes to the chapter
Some names in this chapter have been changed.

Carren Strock was raised by parents who encouraged creativity. She is equally at home with a paintbrush and canvas, needle and thread, or hammer and nails. Luckily, she didn't listen to her college professor who told her that she wasn't a writer. While she is best known for her groundbreaking book *Married Women Who Love Women*, now in its third edition, she is as eclectic in her writing as in her other pursuits. Her books include *A Writer's Journey: What to Know Before, During, and After Writing a Book*, *In the Shadow of the Wonder Wheel* (a mystery novel set in Coney Island, New York; she is currently working on a sequel), *Tangled Ribbons* (a lesbian paranormal romance), *Grandpa and Me and the Park in the City* (a rhyming picture book for children), *Potatoes With Appeal: 105 Mouth-Watering Recipes* (a cookbook) and *Secret Survivors* (a gripping middle-grade chapter book). www.carrenstrock.com

9

Menopause and Transition

Journalist and freelance writer **Lee Hurley** discusses the shock of his journey into menopause as a trans man and explores what menopause means as you move through the landscape of gender, relationships, sex and parenthood.

Menopause, natural or induced, was never something I really thought about. Defined simply as 'the time when there have been no menstrual periods for twelve consecutive months and no other biological or physiological cause can be identified' (on MedicineNet), it eventually happens naturally in those born with ovaries and a womb and is induced in women who wish to transition to male. As I began my transition and was pushed into an induced menopause, via injections and surgery, I still paid it little to no heed. I was more concerned about the second puberty I was going through, all the operations I had to face and the pressure of transitioning socially. I wanted to know when the hair on my face would finally grow. I wanted all the side-effects of menopause that are viewed as a downside: the end to periods, the extra body hair some women get, the vaginal atrophy, so my body stopped producing what had always seemed to me as an excess of lubricant in that area. Nobody at the gender clinic I was obligated to attend for therapy talked about menopause either, at least not in any significant way. It was glossed over as if it was a side-effect of transitioning, like a little too much wind; nothing to worry about and it will soon pass. There is a notion that if you're a trans guy who starts testosterone then the only symptom of menopause you will experience will be the cessation of periods. That made sense. I got an oestrogen blocker after I started testosterone: given in that order, I was told, to stop any menopausal symptoms. Now my transition is complete, it's clear that was not true, but going through a second puberty, menopause, surgeries and everything else all at once, it's hard to know what is causing what at the time.

Looking back over my 'female' life, there's a consistent theme. I didn't know I was trans, but I always found myself turning away from anything seen as feminine or female – clothes, haircuts – I could have gone on the pill to ease my menstrual nightmare, but my brain wouldn't let me go to the doctor to ask for it. I didn't know why; I just knew I didn't want something women took to stop themselves getting pregnant. When being prepped to start testosterone, I was sent for a scan of my reproductive bits. The doctor found large cysts on my ovaries, which he said were probably responsible for my period troubles. If I'd been willing to let anyone, particularly a doctor, near that area, I might have found that out years before. But I wasn't.

By the time my lower surgeries came around, I'd been on testosterone long enough to believe that I was going to be menopause-free. But after surgery it became clear that the blocker had not stopped as much oestrogen flowing through my system as I believed. My then girlfriend, whom I'd met after I started hormones but before lower surgery, commented that I smelled different after I'd had all my internal bits removed. My pee was more manly than before, a common side-effect of testosterone (and why men's public bathrooms smell so bad).

The hormones and surgery all served to push me into a medically induced menopause, but nobody told me that would or could happen. My lower surgery was done in three stages, the most major coming during the second, when they removed everything and stitched everything else up. That's when my ovaries, womb, tubes and everything else were whipped out and they sealed what had been a vagina opening after they removed that part, too. I hadn't had hot sweats before this, but was now regularly waking up so drenched I needed to dry myself off with a towel and change the sheets and pillows. Was it something I'd eaten? Had I had a drink and it was a reaction to alcohol? I tried to find a common cause but there didn't seem to be one. Nor was there one for the sudden longing for a child that railroaded me, to such a degree I found it difficult to be around friends and family members with their own kids; a longing that seemed to come from nowhere. My temper rose and I was quick to snap, finding irritation in the littlest things.

Was that menopause or testosterone? Who could tell? Certainly not any of the medical people I had to deal with throughout my transition, that's for sure. So I spoke to another trans guy, one who already had a child from before he started to transition. 'There's the physical and the psychological,' my friend told me. 'And how much harder it is to reconcile the loss of something you never wanted in the first place. "I don't want this! Why am I losing it?" It's worrying and there's no support. Even my cis female partner was uncomfortable talking about it with me,' said my friend.

'I would go through massive waves of vulnerability and softness and emotional sensitivity that would knock me off,' he continued. 'It felt incompatible with how I wanted to be in the world and how I felt about myself. It got too much. I was dreaming of babies. I was crying. I couldn't work out what the longing and the pain was. I ended up talking to a cis female friend who had gone through menopause. She could relate and shared her stories with me, and it became clear it was definitely menopause. It is the last kick, I guess, to get you to have a baby, whether you physically can or not. It must be the hormones' last hurrah.'

When I started testosterone, my periods stopped a month later. My trans friend wasn't so fortunate:

> I began to wonder if god was having a fucking joke because it just wasn't stopping. It took a year and a half and I went through every form of injectable. On T [testosterone], I bled horribly, and it was unpredictable, it was psychologically mental. It smelled funny, as well. There was a lot of abdominal pain, and that can be a sign of menopause. You also have to remember, we're going through puberty and menopause at the same time, so I don't know if that makes it different. It must do.

'If it wasn't for my friend, it would have been much worse,' he continued:

> There I was, isolated and alone and not able to work it out. I needed someone I could talk to who would honour both my physical container and my

being. What she was basically saying was, 'That's all normal, why would it be any different for you?' There was an emotional longing for babies. Cis men have it as well. Talking to some [cis men], you realise that men's longing for kids doesn't stop when their female partners enter menopause and it doesn't really get recognised that they want to be a father. They grieve not being fathers, too. You only ever hear about it when women can't have kids, you don't hear about the man's longing.

Somewhere in the middle of T, I started to look at baby boots. It was ridiculous. I'd see babies in a totally different way, with a genuine longing for them. It was painful and would have me in tears. I couldn't work myself out. I just wanted to smell them and be around them.

For me, it wasn't quite that intense, but it was there.

Trans people accept, with surprising good grace, that to transition and be themselves they usually have to choose between that and being a biological parent (if they aren't already). Sterility as a side-effect comes on the packet when you are transgender. I was asked – once – if I wanted to freeze any eggs before I started to take testosterone. I didn't, because I hadn't thought about the longer-term implications and was impatient to get my transition going, having waited almost a year just to get my first appointment at the clinic. My therapist was happy enough with my brief 'no' that he didn't feel any need to probe further. As much as society has a problem with getting their head around a pregnant trans man, so too do many of the therapists tasked with guiding us through this journey. It feels, at times, that as long as you stick to what are considered traditional cishet norms, you'll keep them happy. Step outside those and suddenly your transition becomes a bit of a hassle: more paperwork, more awkwardness, more hoops to jump through to prove you really are the gender you say you are.

Often, it felt as if some of those who were there to supposedly help were secretly glad we were being made infertile by the process. Perhaps it was the subtle smile I noticed as they quickly moved the subject on, or the transphobic comments some therapists made regularly during sessions that added up to give this impression. Like the one who told me, 'All you trans men look the same,' or the one who told my friend, 'No woman would want a man' with the surgery he was opting for (a metoidioplasty that would result in a fully sensate but micro penis). These are conversations, sadly, that happen often between trans people in private, but they are too afraid to speak of publicly lest they lose access to the treatment they need. Others, however, have taken the NHS in England to court over its failure to provide these services.

Although I cannot father a child, a future partner could have carried one of my eggs, fertilised by a donor, and that, to me now, would have felt as much 'our' biological child as if I'd provided sperm instead. At the very least, I should have been pushed to consider it more. I don't know if I'd have listened, but someone should have pushed. No other options were presented. NHS guidelines even state:

> Hormone therapy will also make both trans men and trans women less fertile and, eventually, completely infertile. Your specialist should discuss the implications for fertility before starting treatment, and they may talk to you about the option of storing eggs or sperm (known as gamete storage) in case you want to have children in the future.

At 36, when I came out as trans, it felt like my fertile time was almost up anyway, but we now have many 17- and 18-year-olds making the same decisions without being pushed to seriously consider the ramifications of their choices further down the line.

'I'd had a child before accepting I was trans because my girlfriend couldn't,' my friend reflected:

> It was never really my plan but more a result of circumstance. I thought, 'OK, I can do this!' I was petrified, but I did it. That's how I know about the hormonal shift the other way – the pregnancy hormones. They are totally and completely different. I became a different person. People just don't understand the power of hormones. That cooking of my brain and pregnancy hormones lasted for years, it changed me mentally.

When you say 'hormones' most people only think about testosterone and oestrogen, but hormones were 'the last major system in the body to be discovered and we're still discovering more all the time', according to John Wass, professor of endocrinology at Oxford University, quoted in Bill Bryson's book *The Body*. Before the end of the 1950s, there were only about twenty hormone chemicals known to science. Now, nobody seems to have a clue how many there are – and they are produced throughout the body, not just in the endocrine glands as traditionally thought. Even your bones and stomach produce hormones. Wass thinks there are at least eighty, possibly 100 hormones. What is clear is that no one can agree and, as all these hormones do different things, come from different places, can be steroids, proteins or amines, they are linked only, Bryson writes, 'by their purpose, not their chemistry. Our understanding of them is far from complete and much of what we do know is surprisingly recent.'

If a clinical trial was proposed that forced people to switch their sex hormones just to study the results, there would rightly be a universal outcry. Thankfully, however, that isn't necessary, because there are plenty of us out there doing it voluntarily and the data that could be collected would astound, if only anyone cared enough to collect it. Or even realise that it's there. Being trans does sometimes feel like being a walking, talking experiment. We are a living, breathing representation of the impact of hormones, a part of us all so important and powerful that we wouldn't – and couldn't – be us without them.

With trans people, there is a chance to study the power of at least two hormones up close and very personally. As I began my transition journey, I remember my friend, Etain O'Kane, a cis female Belfast therapist who used to facilitate trans support groups, saying she had noticed 'the effects of hormone change that challenged [her] assumptions'. She could see 'that certain gendered behaviours were not simply learned or performed, but had a physiological basis'. By removing oestrogen, as much as possible, from my own system, and adding testosterone, I personally felt like my brain had been rewired. I am calmer, more assured and certainly have more confidence. I no longer have wild emotional fluctuations at all, let alone every month. More often than not, I can set emotion aside at will; something that was impossible before. Of course, being able to live as my true self has helped immensely in terms of my confidence, and this is far from a controlled experiment, but now that my hormones feel more aligned to a way of being in the world that is natural to me, I see more rationally and am able to control (or gain perspective on) my emotions, something that was impossible before. That's leaving aside the physical changes which are obvious to everyone – the broader shoulders, the deeper voice, the big ginger beard. Sadly, I can also report that a lot of what we want to believe are gender stereotypes, dictated by society, also from my experience seem to be driven by these particular hormones.

It's common, for example, to think that men don't cry because we raise boys to be tough, and that's true. To an extent. But testosterone also makes it physically harder to cry and every transitioning trans man I've spoken to says the same. It's a common discussion point among us, especially at the start of our transition. Previously, when I was O-fuelled, I cried all the time. It was frustrating as hell. I couldn't stop and that just made it more frustrating. My body's reaction to that? More tears. I had trouble controlling my emotions, and always felt like an irrational teenager who hadn't quite managed to get a hold of things during puberty (or escape it for twenty-five years). I hated it all and found it incredibly embarrassing.

Then I changed to T. About a year later, the man I loved more than any other lay dying an agonising death and I both wanted and desperately needed to let that emotion out. I couldn't for the longest time. No tears would come, no matter how much I tried to open myself to them. When they eventually fell, they poured from my eyes like a torrential downpour, the pain reaching depths that only grief can touch, and then they stopped. Quickly. There was no lingering or extended crying sessions. There was no curling up in a ball on the bed, unable to face the world because I couldn't stop myself from crying, and I knew that's exactly how I would have been before.

I am acutely aware of not making a chapter on menopause all about men. We have a tendency to do that with everything else, but whether it's uncomfortable for you or not, some men have bits that mean they not only bleed every month like cis women, they also face the prospect of menopause, too. And a man is, unfortunately, what I am, even though I wasn't endowed with those biological bits when I came into this world at someone else's behest. Trust me, I'd much rather be this happy and still a lesbian – men are mostly dicks – but that was not possible. I know because I spent twenty-five years trying to make it so.

For trans men, menopause is both the start of something and the end. For cis women it is the same, but as a society we don't tend to view it that way. Instead of ushering in a sense of freedom and a signal that this is the time for 'you', we tell postmenopausal people ... well, nothing really, because they just stop existing in so many ways. The most I hear about menopause is people talking about hot flushes and then women laughing together, but nobody seems to talk about it at any deeper level, or what any of it means. Should it be mourned, or celebrated, or both? 'I guess maybe it depends on if you have kids or not, because at least you have something,' my friend said, before also pointing out that we are now no different to cis guys having to rely on a woman to carry a baby.

'I was talking to a woman about attitudes to fathers,' he added:

She was talking about how women won the right to financial freedom; we don't need men for anything, ha! And I pointed out men also won the right to have their own kids and bring them up. It's a two-way thing. Both are burdened, but the female attitude to men as fathers seems to be you either get a patronising 'Aww god love you, you're doing so well,' which is a bit mucky but quite nice, or, 'You're a hero.' Every single parent is a hero, end of story. But there is a constant pervasive message that you're not doing it right because it's not to 'female' standards. As a perceived butch woman, it was demeaning – 'You're not up to scratch, love, because you're butch and your methods are different.' Now, I get the same thing but also a horrible bitterness as well.

Being trans took up a lot of my brainspace, leaving little room to think of other things or cope with life in general. It was only when I got to the other side of that journey that I was able to exist in any meaningful way, and to start thinking of those things – like if I might like to have a child in the not-too-distant future. By then, however, it was too late. You also have to deal with a lot of transphobia, both internal and external. 'If society had less prejudice towards trans people, stopped calling us freaks or broken,' he added, 'it would be totally different. But it's not like that now. Even I find the sight of a pregnant trans man peculiar. It's a step braver than ever before. The support you need when you are pregnant ... to miss out on all that is awful.'

I wanted to find a trans woman who could talk to me about their experience: about the subject of menopause and attitudes towards them as older women. I contacted a few trans women I know personally but got no reply. I set up a questionnaire so it could be discussed anonymously, and I got one half-filled-out reply from a trans guy. I asked on Facebook and Twitter, where I have a decent following and major trans accounts retweeted my plea. Still, no one appeared to want to talk.

That's totally understandable. Menopause, like periods, is seen as such an intrinsically 'female' thing, that even just discussing it brings up feelings of being 'different' and, perhaps, in some instances, 'not being woman enough'. Of course, there are also cis women who don't experience menopause, those who had their ovaries removed during childhood, before puberty, for instance. Yet it is seen as such a universal female experience, asking trans women to discuss it is asking them to open up about a longing perhaps they aren't quite ready to face. I know that's what writing this chapter has done for me.

I braced myself and hit Google. There, mostly I found cis women complaining that trans men were being included in any moves in employment law to make accommodation for those going through menopause. 'The struggle for women to get recognition of the often-debilitating effects of the menopause has long been ridiculed and just as it starts to be taken seriously, it appears to be subsumed into the current clamour to be all-inclusive, even at the apparent exclusion of how some women might feel,' wrote Mandy Rhodes, editor of *Holyrood*, in 2019.

Unlike the usual discussion around trans people, where trans men are all too often forgotten about, in this one, it seems, it is trans women who are ignored. Menstrual symptoms, however, are often present in trans women who transition, but as menopause is the cessation of the production of oestrogen, continuing to receive regular oestrogen boosters should stave off most effects.

Dr Helen Webberley, the founder of the online transgender clinic GenderGP, which supports trans and non-binary individuals around the world with their health and well-being needs, told me:

Reaching menopausal age as a trans woman brings with it a whole new set of questions. Should the individual be slowly weaned off their hormones, to mirror the natural process of a cis woman? What would be the impact? Would the feminising effects experienced to date be reversed? Would testosterone levels start to rise or, given that testosterone levels reduce with age in cis men, is this no longer a concern? Is it safer to be free of the effects of oestrogen due to the increased risk of blood clots and breast cancer or should one continue on hormones given the perceived benefits for heart and bone health?

This shows that much is yet to be learned on menopause in all people and while uncertainty exists, it's important to take into account what we do know from a medical perspective, alongside the wishes and expectations of the individual. The psychological impact of stopping hormones on the individual should not be underestimated; hormones can positively affect the way the individual sees themselves and the ways in which they believe they are perceived by society.

All this, and I haven't even touched on non-binary and intersex people.

In short, hormones, and everything we think of as 'female' or 'male', is up for grabs and while we can point to a majority experiencing certain conditions, we can no longer say anything is solely the domain of one gender or another. Not that there are only two genders, just like there are not only two sexualities, shapes of ears, noses, heads, bodies, colours of eyes, hair, height or build.

After being asked to write this chapter, I flung the word menopause around in my head. I battered it against old memories and pushed it into dark and dusty corners, in search of any evidence of how and when it featured in my thirty-six-year life as a woman. There was little to be found. I did remember a life with a reproductive system that felt as if it had been trying to kill me since I had my first period, aged 10, and a desire for that hell to stop. If menopause featured in my thinking at all, that's what it was to me: an end to the severe monthly pain and the six or seven migraines with it. The bleeding was so heavy I'd go through the most absorbent tampons in an hour and a half, afraid to leave the house in case I leaked everywhere. Pads never felt like an option.

I also never wanted to be pregnant. That never seemed like it would feel right. Even as a 21-year-old lesbian, madly in love with a partner I wanted to have kids with, when we talked about it, it was her who would carry them. What if she couldn't, she asked me? I knew I was lying as I said of course I would.

Now, at least, I no longer have to lie about any of it. Menopause, then, if it was anything to me, was freedom from the last remnants of my old self and the start of my new life as me.

Lee Hurley is a freelance writer who lives and works in Belfast. He started to transition from female to male in 2012 and has written for a number of well-known publications, including the *Guardian* and *Vice*, on the topic of being a transgender man while also running a football site. This probably makes him the only professional sports writer in the world who is a trans guy. Now 44 yet also just coming out of another puberty, Lee lives alone with his adorable, but dramatic, dog.

10

A Cellular Experience

Writer **Clare Barstow** explores how her time in prison exposed her to the harrowing lack of provision for and understanding of women's health in the UK criminal justice system. Her experiences shed light on an often neglected area of menopause care.

Prison as a punishment is supposed to entail purely the loss of freedom as its main objective. However, the impact that a long period of incarceration has on your health can't be underestimated. The prison healthcare system provides a very basic service and is ill equipped to deal with women's needs. As women make up only 5 per cent of the prison population their issues are often overlooked. Menopause in particular isn't taken seriously and currently women in the criminal justice system do not have the same access to care as that provided in the community, which is the recommendation of Public Health England in its 2018 report 'Gender Specific Standards to Improve Health and Well-being for Women in Prison in England'.

I first started noticing a change in my menstrual cycle when I was 50 and had been in prison for twenty years. I had always suffered long, painful and heavy periods but they seemed to be getting worse and much more frequent. I would wake up in the morning and discover that I had bled through my night clothes and all the sheets. The prison frequently ran out of sanitary towels and tampons so I wouldn't always have any spare. Also, women would use sanitary towels to clean the cell floor, as the cleaning materials were woefully inadequate. We were only allowed one set of sheets a week – a problem also highlighted by the Prison Reform Trust in its 2008 report 'Doing Time: The Experiences and Needs of Older People in Prison'. We would have to change them in the prison laundry, so most women washed them by hand as the embarrassment of queuing up on a Friday with blood-stained sheets was often too much to bear. In prisons, an Incentives and Earned Privileges (IEP) scheme has operated since 1995. When you first come into prison you are on the Standard regime. Systems vary between prisons, but where I was, after eight weeks, if you had three positive entries on your file, then you could be moved up to the Enhanced level (likewise, if you had three negative entries you could be moved down to Basic). If you get to Enhanced, you can buy your own sheets – but only if you are lucky enough to have money sent in. Even then you can only wash them once a week in the laundry, so you aren't much better off.

In my prison, you couldn't access effective painkillers as only paracetamol was issued, so often you had to work in incredible pain and would feel exhausted and drained all the time. The humiliation of constantly bleeding through your clothes meant that many women were scared to socialise and preferred to get an adjudication as well as a punishment for not going to work, rather than be laughed at by fellow prisoners and staff alike. (An adjudication is when you break a prison rule and have to appear before a governor to explain yourself; if found guilty, you are punished by being locked up more of the time, for example, or losing the chance to buy necessities from the prison shop.) There were no support services such as regular access to counselling, and even though I was on a healthcare focus group and would argue for changes, these groups achieved very little and in my experience were usually a tick-box exercise. I would witness girls in tears as they were in such pain and were so demoralised by their treatment.

Healthcare in English prisons is currently commissioned by NHS England Health and Justice and, in a substantial number, key elements of the healthcare service are outsourced to private contractors. These companies then become responsible for the quality of the healthcare provision in prison. This was the case where I was imprisoned, and meant that if you were receiving poor treatment, you had to complain to the contractor. I found that they took a long time to investigate and the responses were often cursory. As they had to aim to make a profit, it meant a reduction in specialist services and cutbacks, leading to a very basic quality of care. I was released from prison in 2017, but more recently released women say nothing has changed in the effectiveness of the healthcare service.

Women in the criminal justice system have much more serious health issues than in the general population, due to a history of complex needs from experiences of abject poverty, domestic abuse, substance misuse, psychological trauma or other negative factors – as noted in Public Health England's report on standards for women in prison. According to the campaigning organisation Women in Prison, over 60 per cent of women in contact with the criminal justice system have experienced domestic abuse, 53 per cent of women in prison have experienced physical, sexual or psychological trauma during childhood and 31 per cent of women in prison have experienced time in local authority care as a child. There is also prejudice against Black, Asian and Minority Ethnic (BAME) prisoners; for example, if they are suffering with mental health issues these can get mislabelled as anger management issues. The Lammy Report of 2017, 'Double Disadvantage', spoke to BAME women in focus groups who said that if they associated in groups it was often seen as a gang and that they were dealing prison medication, whereas their white counterparts didn't suffer from the same perception issues.

The female prison population is getting increasingly older. In the UK, there has been a 150 per cent increase between 2002 and 2017 in the proportion of people aged 50 or over in prison, according to Public Health England. For myself, I slowly started noticing changes in my mental and physical health. I am normally a pretty balanced person as I have been a Buddhist for thirty years, but then I realised I was suffering from irrational mood swings and was prone to tears. I began to get hot flushes and felt sick. Then the dizzy spells started and I kept on fainting, eventually injuring myself when I fell. When I spoke about this, the male doctors showed little sympathy and refused to sign me off from work, even though I could barely walk. I had to sleep in sweat-ridden sheets for a week in the summer, as there was no heating to dry them on. I ended up in a wheelchair several times, due to constantly falling over.

Even though I told the healthcare staff I was going through the menopause, they refused to test me and my condition was seen as a mental health issue. I had to explain to a psychologist what the matter was, but again nothing was done. Female prisoners are labelled as doubly damned and doubly devious because society perceives that as a woman, mother, carer, wife you have to be perfect and are therefore twice as bad if you commit a crime. This means you are not taken seriously, and it is assumed you are making everything up. There were many other women going through the same traumas as me, but the healthcare service refused to listen.

Public Health England's 'Gender Specific Standards to Improve Health and Well-being for Women in Prison in England' details the range of support that should be offered to older women, which they admit is not being met. These measures include specific screening for older women upon entering prison and then every six months. In my experience, and from what I have seen and heard from other women, this doesn't happen. Most of the recommendations for older women have not been implemented, including help for women with the menopause, as women who recently left prison have confirmed.

In the end I was so sick with the effect the menopause was having on my body that I had to call the Listeners, who are fellow prisoners trained by the Samaritans. I had been one myself in the past and I knew that if the staff were neglecting me, they might be able to help. I was so dehydrated and exhausted that I started hallucinating. Being constantly sick and inconti- nent meant that my body was in meltdown. When the Listeners witnessed how bad I was, they reported it to Safer Custody, a department within the prison which deals with the safeguarding of prisoners. I went to hospital the next day. I had ended up with a urinary tract infection. I told the doctor at the hospital everything that had happened and he sent a letter on my release from hospital back to the prison, recommending I be given HRT to stop the constant fainting and falling over.

Eventually, after a few weeks, when the tests came back, I was given a course of HRT tablets. However, even then it wasn't smooth, as the prison pharmacy frequently ran out of tablets. I had to order them monthly a week before they ran out, but even then I would turn up to collect them and they wouldn't be there. It sometimes took a week for the HRT to arrive, so the impact on my body of constantly being on or off the tablets was pretty hor- rendous. This was also the experience of others on tablets, and women who were on HRT patches had the same problem. Then the pharmaceutical com- pany stopped manufacturing my tablets and I had to wait several weeks for a different brand.

With HRT there can also be a problem with breakthrough bleeding, which means you can bleed at any time. This meant I had to wear sanitary protection all the time. As there was such a shortage of sanitary towels, I ended up asking the doctor for incontinence pads, as at least I could then have protection theoretically all the time. However, these were issued on a very ad hoc basis and often the incontinence nurse didn't have any or couldn't be reached. I was also getting stress incontinence and my menopausal symptoms exacerbated this.

I started going through menopause in a prison where I had to share a room. This was incredibly humiliating when it came to the regular heavy periods and the incontinence, as I often stained the bed and was doubly ashamed that my roommate saw it. She didn't understand as she was younger than me and got quite upset with me. We also had to share the showers and could only access these at certain times – so any hope of a midnight shower to release the night sweats was impossible. I found it incredibly difficult not having any privacy while going through such a life-changing experience. I also had to try to keep my emotions in check, as I didn't want any conflicts to arise. It was like keeping a lid on Pandora's box. Other older women would cry as they were so embarrassed by their symptoms.

Some of the women came from cultures where periods were seen as dirty and they couldn't talk about the menopause or what they were suffering as it was considered unwomanly. A friend who I worked with suffered even more extremes of agony, as she had gone through very invasive female genital mutilation (FGM), which meant that not only had her clitoris been removed but her vagina had been partially sewn up, so she was in agony every time she had her period or went to the toilet. Luckily, she confided in me and I was able to persuade her to go to the doctors for help. At least the HRT seemed to mitigate her symptoms slightly.

Working for most of my sentence in the library meant that I had access to health information on a regular basis, but most of the women didn't have this luxury. I was also able to suggest different titles for the librarian to order. The budget was extremely limited and seemed to get cut every year, but we were able to order a couple of books about the menopause. The trouble was they quickly became out of date in a few years, as new research brought increased understanding about the menopause. However, there was no new money to keep the books up to date, so often they were up to ten years old. It was the same with a lot of the health section.

We did have an over-fifties group in the prison I was in, but the supposed monthly meetings were often cancelled. Some of us raised our concerns about how the menopause was affecting our daily lives, but as the health-care service rarely attended these meetings nothing concrete was done. Again, it was just a tick-box exercise to show they met diversity require-ments. I was also on the Diversity Committee, but hardly any attention was paid to female health issues as most of the staff who attended were male. Many women found it embarrassing to raise so-called women's issues in front of men in particular.

A friend of mine spoke with me about her experience of going through the menopause in a different prison and she found it incredibly tough. She didn't understand what a hot flush was and thought something dreadful was happening. She struggled a huge amount with not having access to clean bedding. This only added to her anxiety and mental health problems. The healthcare service promised a special menopause clinic, but it never materialised. She felt isolated and alone, which caused her mental health to deteriorate dramatically. Her Asian background meant she felt unable to confide in others about what she was going through and the male doc-tors thought she was exaggerating her condition. She also struggled with weight gain, which is a massive problem for all women in prison.

The diet where I was in prison was incredibly poor and there were few options to purchase healthy food from the prison shop. This meant many women were left feeling depressed about a weight gain they could do nothing about. The lack of good nutrition and balanced meals meant that many struggled to stay healthy. As a vegetarian, I had real problems with my weight, and other health issues meant I spent time immobile, which just added to already serious health conditions. The Public Health England guidelines draw on a report from the National Audit Office, 'Serving Time: Prisoner Diet and Exercise' (2006), to comment that:

Many of the meals examined were high in calories, and these exceeded government recommendations, and were also high in saturated fatty acids. Many of these meals relied heavily on convenience foods such as pies and burgers and tinned food, with little use of seasonal produce.

Gym provision in the female establishment is much poorer than for the men, as a patriarchal system considers women to be less interested in sport and therefore in need of less physical exercise – something that has been confirmed to me by gym officers who have worked in both male and female establishments. All this despite the proven physical and mental benefits of regular exercise. The over-35s gym that I attended was often cancelled as they simply didn't have the staff to run it. And even though you could have your weight measured, it wasn't monitored regularly enough. There was also a lack of educational funding for healthy living and nutrition courses, as education wasn't viewed to be as important for women as for men. Many of the classes were very basic and there was a distinct lack of funding for anything worthwhile. While many men have access to full-time education, this certainly wasn't true for women in the prison I have experience of, who struggled to get on courses that had huge waiting lists.

The other trouble with weight gain is you only get paid £10 a week, so you can't afford to buy new clothes all the time. You also have to wait ages for any order of prison-issue clothes from the stores department. As you had to work in these, you couldn't keep them clean, so you were walking around in dirty clothes – which also added to the depression. If you were lucky you had family or friends outside who might send you in money to buy clothes, but many women didn't have this luxury. There are also the added health risks associated with weight gain. These could be more life-threatening in prison than in the community, owing to the poor healthcare and the length of time it took to arrange hospital appointments, which were always being cancelled due to lack of staff.

Osteoporosis was also a really serious and common health condition among the women in prison. Yvonne Jewkes and her co-authors in the *Handbook on Prisons* state that women are three to five times more likely to have hip, back and spine impairments than men due to osteoporosis. I encountered a lot of women with osteoporosis who had difficulty getting enough calcium, vitamin D and medication. They were supposed to be allocated extra milk, but this often wasn't there when they went to pick it up. The lack of outdoor exercise and sunlight contributed to many women having seriously low levels of vitamin D. I myself was eventually, after a few months, diagnosed with a lack of vitamin D and as a result had to take tablets. Often, again, the tablets weren't there when I went to collect them, which led to a reduction in their effectiveness. Bone fractures as a result of osteoporosis were common and sometimes they wouldn't be diagnosed as fractures for a long time, leading to serious mobility issues further down the line. BAME women in particular suffer from reduced vitamin D and this is only exacerbated by the menopause and the much higher risk of osteoporosis. The women I knew who had osteoporosis were usually from BAME backgrounds, yet they weren't given regular health check-ups. In the community, yearly check-ups are pretty standard if you have an existing health condition and are on medication, but not in the prison system, so many health conditions can become more serious through lack of care and lead to other illnesses not being identified in time.

Lack of sleep was also very problematic, as being locked in a cell with few distractions, compounded by insomnia, had drastic effects on the well-being of the women. The tiredness affected their mood and their inability to perform daily tasks effectively, including work, often led to them being disciplined by the staff. You could be given warnings as part of the IEP scheme, which could result in you losing Enhanced or Standard status and you could end up on the Basic regime. This meant you were locked in your cell most of the time without a television, which resulted in more mental health issues. This happened to me, as I was too sick to work but didn't get a proper diagnosis for over a year. Most women struggled to get any sleeping medication from the healthcare service as the doctors didn't understand the issues they had. You only had ten minutes with the doctor, so you never had time to explain all the added difficulties you were facing.

Loss of hair and dry skin as symptoms of the menopause were more of an issue in prison, as the poor diet made things worse. Also, you couldn't access or afford to buy any products that would help with these and – from what I witnessed and heard about – the doctors wouldn't prescribe anything. Some prisons had hairdressing salons which allowed the women to be trained there. However, there were huge waiting lists and many women couldn't afford to pay. Alopecia was common, as the added stress of confinement only exacerbated the problem. Dry skin often led to more serious rashes and skin diseases were relatively common.

Joint pains, headaches and other aches and pains as a result of the menopause are a real issue, due to lack of access to effective painkillers. The doctors were reluctant to give anything stronger than paracetamol as some women had issues with drug addiction, but they should have examined each case individually rather than going for a blanket ban. The healthcare service was supposed to be a trauma-informed enabling environment, but this was far from the case. Many women found it to be the most distressing encounter of their prison sentence and some were forced to make complaints to the private contractor who was responsible for healthcare provision. I had to have several meetings with the contractor and even engaged an outside advocate as well as a prison law solicitor before my situation was finally resolved. Fortunately, I was educated enough to fight my case, but many didn't because they couldn't write or were too scared of repercussions.

The lack of regular clinics was also an issue. A gynaecologist rarely came to the establishment so many serious issues weren't diagnosed in time. A doctor told me that I had fibroids, but I wasn't taken to hospital to see a specialist (this was the case for many women) until the fibroids became too large and had to be operated on. Hysterectomies cause very severe physical and psychological problems for women in prison, according to Yvonne Jewkes in the *Handbook on Prisons*. Access to physiotherapy could be patchy and the Well Woman Clinic was often cancelled due to lack of staff. Smear tests were infrequent, and the lack of diagnosis could have serious consequences. Nadia Escobar and Emma Plugge wrote about this in an article in *The Journal of Epidemiology and Community Health* from October 2019, in which they recorded their findings that the rates of invasive cervical cancer in prisons in the UK, US and Canada were 100 times higher than in the community. Cervical cancer screening rates in the UK were also sixteen times higher in the community than in prison. From my experience, regular breast screening didn't take place, due to a lack of staff for escorts and failures in administration. My last one was two years late. The pain clinic rarely happened, and many women suffered unnecessarily.

Many women couldn't speak English or couldn't write, so without a translator no one knew what they were suffering. If help had been provided, they might not have had to go through menopause without any support. A lack of cultural understanding and marginalisation were common factors in the failure to diagnose menopause and other health issues. For the Travelling Community, an absence of formal education meant they were scared to seek help when needing to fill out an application to see the healthcare service. The problem was that you had to apply for everything, so if you couldn't read or write, then your chances of being seen by the healthcare service or being able to communicate what your needs were would be pretty low. Even though I helped a lot of women fill out forms, there were many who were left undiagnosed as a result of there being no specialised provision.

The effect of the menopause on women's mental health mustn't be underestimated. One lady in her fifties was suffering really badly with the side-effects, but no one would listen to her. The constant mood swings were making her extremely depressed and she ended up self-harming badly. Tragically, the woman died as a result of this self-harming, and she was not an isolated case. Self-harm is particularly high in the female estate and lack of effective health provision is often a triggering point. The Ministry of Justice Safer Custody statistics for the year up to March 2019 state there are 2,828 self-harming incidents for every 1,000 women, an increase of 22 per cent on the previous year.

As a Listener, I witnessed so many older women struggling with the menopause and not being taken seriously. I heard a number of male staff laughing in the office, being dismissive of women and their suffering, saying, 'It's only the menopause', which was derogatory and diminishing. Despite a formal complaint about this, no action was taken.

Anxiety causes major trauma for most women and for some this is worsened by the menopause. Some women become so anxious they are scared to go out from their cell. It also induces paranoia. One lady became seriously anorexic rather than have to go to the dining room and face people. Confusion is the hardest thing – when women don't understand what is happening to their bodies and they think they are going mad. Being locked away only compounds this, but the hormonal imbalance could be rectified if only they were taken seriously.

Access to natural remedies as alternatives to HRT are virtually non-existent too. One of the prisoners on a herbalism course started giving the women sage to counteract the symptoms. However, if you were caught with this in your cell you could be punished as a result. The healthcare service in my prison was very narrow-minded when it came to alternative therapies.

So, what could be done to really improve the treatment of menopausal women in the criminal justice system? Specific focus groups should be held within the female establishments to ensure clarity and for feedback. The women who take part need to be chosen from diverse backgrounds to ensure true representation. Questionnaires could be put under everyone's doors to allow other women to have a say. Leaflets with information on the menopause could also be put under every door. Menopause clinics should be held as a matter of course in all the healthcare departments. The Ministry of Justice and National Health England need to be made aware of the problems women face in accessing vital aspects of the health services. The private contractors who deliver healthcare in female prisons need to have special provision set up for specialist needs such as the menopause. Groups and charities could be invited in to talk about women's health issues, including menopause. Prison staff should be given special training to understand the condition and how it might affect the women in their care. Probation staff should also undergo a course on this subject.

The *Prison Service Instructions* are a set of rules, regulations and guidelines upon which prisons are run. These need to have better instructions looking at female health needs. This could allow for more sanitary protection, regular access to the washing machines or prison laundry, access to different clothing sizes for prison issue and personal purchase, extra clothing, more exercise opportunities including tailor-made individual programmes (particularly for clients with osteoporosis), translation services for those who can't understand English, access to better pain relief and more female doctors, among other helpful requirements. A specially trained Menopause Champion in each prison would also be appreciated, as they could ensure all the women's needs were being met. Unless the criminal justice system starts taking the menopause seriously as a health condition, many more women will suffer needlessly.

Clare Barstow was born in Kent and studied Classics and Ancient History at Royal Holloway College, University of London. She took a diploma in Journalism at the London College of Printing before working at various publishers on a variety of magazines including *Tatler*, *Music Week*, *Travel Bulletin* and *Care Weekly*. After six years she went freelance and contributed to everything from *Chat*, *Bella* and *TV Quick* to *Campaign* and *School Leaver* as a journalist and sub-editor. More recently, she has worked at *Inside Times* and *The View* magazine. Clare was sent to prison for murder in 1992, but always maintained her innocence and ended up serving a much longer sentence as a result. She also writes plays and has had several performed in various theatres around the world. As an artist, she has recently worked on a series concerning female genital mutilation (FGM) and has had her work exhibited regularly. Her interest in medical matters comes from her brother being a doctor and her father working in the pharmaceutical industry.

11

A Flâneuse of This Sickness

Cat Chong is a poet in their twenties, who is also a PhD student in Medical Humanities at Nanyang Technological University (NTU) in Singapore. They explore how we use language to frame the menopause and reflect in conversation on society's difficult relationship with the female body from a non-binary perspective.

> I typed into the Google Doc at 4 am, 'menopause turns females into dandies'.
>
> Lisa Robertson, *Proverbs of a She-Dandy*

When I think about menopause, initially I see it as a physically uncomfortable inheritance, an experience that I may have to undergo either as a young person due to illness, or as someone older due to time. As I write this, I am 22, disabled, and a non-binary woman; my relationship to menopause is a complicated one. In *Proverbs of a She-Dandy*, Lisa Robertson explores the figure of the flâneur: typically a male character; someone who dandies, who wanders or strolls through a city or other environment, pausing at and noting points of interest, as we might do when visitors in another culture or when seeing our own afresh. Robertson considers the way in which menopause can grant women a different form of agency and so acknowledge the presence of the older woman in public spaces. I would like to take the position of a flâneuse to consider how menopause can occur in younger bodies, and how this affects my own relationship with the normative image of the menopausal woman. I wish to dandy, I wish to wander in and explore the landscape of endometriosis, age and womanhood.

It has been over a year since I've had a period, and four years since I began taking contraceptive pills back-to-back in order to prevent them. I have never menstruated regularly; my body resolved at an early age to avoid the formal introduction to regular cycles of blood loss. While attending what was, for a long time, the only British international school in Singapore, I had four periods a year: one during each holiday. Stress, pressure and anxiety prevented the rest of them. Like many of the girls in my cohort, I was also anaemic – as we discovered, in a darkly comic fashion, during an unsuccessful attempt at blood donation. In April of 2019 I had an intrauterine system fitted, otherwise known as an IUS, meaning that I will, for the next three years, experience a complete cessation of periods. An IUS is similar to the intrauterine device (IUD), but instead of releasing copper like the IUD, it releases the hormone progestogen into the womb. Having an IUS was my response to the agony that was induced by menstruation; an agony that is one of the hallmark experiences of endometriosis.

Seven and a half years recuperating a name

According to the Royal College of Nursing endometriosis fact sheet, 'one in 10 women of reproductive age in the UK suffer from endometriosis'. It is, they say, the second most common gynaecological condition in the UK, after fibroids. Like many, I was at first incorrectly treated for irritable bowel syndrome (IBS) and while I still don't have a diagnosis for my own chronic pain condition, I share many symptoms with those who have endometriosis.

The long, polysyllabic, almost agglutinative quality of medical terms is not unfamiliar to me. When I was a child, rather than twist my tongue around the nonsensical nursery rhymes that appeared in my favourite films – the family constant being the *Singin' in the Rain* (1952) variation of 'Moses supposes his toeses are roses, but Moses supposes erroneously ...'

– I would memorise the ever-changing diagnoses ascribed to my mother's chronic illnesses. I could spell 'systemic lupus erythematosus' by the age of 10; my mother, herself an ex-nurse, taught me to detangle and decipher each segment in turn. The same could be said of 'myalgic encephalomyelitis', which I had learned by the age of 12; terms like 'fibromyalgia' and 'chronic fatigue syndrome' seemed simple by comparison. Many diagnostic labels have Greek or Latin roots and often describe the part of the body they affect. Naming – being able to claim a condition with medical authority – means having access to treatment, to financial aid, to visibility, to support networks, to care and the care of others.

Endometriosis is no different and is comprised of three Greek words: εντός (entós) meaning inside, it is the Greek preposition for 'in' or 'within'; μήτρα (mítra) meaning womb, the Greek stem word referring to the uterus; and νόσος (nósos) meaning disease, medically denoting disease as a state, this word is formed from the aorist of verbs ending in -o.

I didn't know what 'aorist' meant so I looked it up in the *Oxford English Dictionary*.

aorist, *n.*
Etymology: < Greek ἀόριστος indefinite, < ἀ priv. + ὁριστός, < ὁρίζειν to limit, define.

In classical Greek, 'aorist' can indicate a past action without reference to whether the action involved is momentary or continuous. It's a nuance that, while clear in Greek, is not commonly used in English. I was surprised how apt this seemed in relation to endometriosis as well as menopause; the onset of the condition being in the past tense but without any reference to having passed to completion. It is a condition that is defined by its duration and subjectivity; both momentary and continuous.

On average it takes seven and a half years from the onset of symptoms of endometriosis to diagnosis. This is according to the Royal College of Nursing; the 13,500 women who took part in BBC research in 2019 recorded the same number: 'In the UK it takes an average of 7.5 years to be diagnosed.' I know I still have longer to wait before I reach a diagnosis of any kind. I too am in a liminal state with no reference to completion. I am in constant pain and periods only make it worse, they involve mood swings, discomfort, and a certain level of gender dysphoria. As someone who is starting to adopt a non-binary identity, I am more comfortable in a body that doesn't menstruate. Sometimes I think I would be more comfortable in a postmenopausal one.

In negotiating this experience of pain and patience as a young person, menopause rushes into the foreground for those with endometriosis, as hormonally induced or surgical menopause is sometimes offered as a form of treatment. While I've been on contraceptives for a number of years, and pain management medication too, for me, menopause discussions have never taken place within a doctor's office. Instead they have occupied living rooms, kitchens, bedrooms, with friends and a warm cup of tea, locating menopause as a domestic rather than medical affair.

Speaking with a friend

Many of my best friends are women whose bodies also refuse to comply with normative modes of being; we share experiences and problems, and I often ask them for advice. The NHS, pain and womanhood are complicated and challenging systems to navigate – being able to learn from and offer solidarity to one another has been invaluable. To me, this slow in-gathering of information between us acts as a feminist demonstration of the notion of council: an assembly of advisors collectivising menopause within young AFAB (assigned female at birth) bodies, organised along the lines of sickness and discomfort.

When speaking with my friend Paige, whose responses counterpoint mine through these following pages, I will never forget the immediate 'no' she pronounced when I inquired after her opinion on induced menopause. I asked her what it was like and she said simply: 'Hell'.

I didn't know that it would be so different from menopause that occurred naturally with age. Paige explained:

I think the big difference is the suddenness. For my mother, menopause came on slowly, as it generally does. Hot flashes etc. For me it kicked in pretty much overnight. I thought I was going mad. Also awful because a lot of it mimics pregnancy, which I wanted so badly – so I thought I was both losing it and pregnant and dying.

My own opiate withdrawal symptoms were very similar to the sudden menopause process that Paige was talking about and I was surprised that they were so alike, that menopause had been an experience for Paige like withdrawal was for me. I wanted to think about this, how opiate withdrawal might allow me to dandy within menopause, to wander coincidentally into the same experience from an utterly different pathway. I was prescribed multiple types of painkillers as part of pain management for my own condition. Over the course of two years, I was given increasingly stronger narcotics – highly addictive and with horrendous side-effects – until I found myself barely able to function. This changed in the summer of 2018, when an abrupt note from a specialist informed me in austere terms that she could do nothing else for me but untether me from her care while on the strongest opiates available. It felt and read like a medical break-up text and was by far the most devastating break-up I've had to date. I made a desperate and, with hindsight, reckless decision to go 'cold turkey' during that summer before I began my MA course.

It took almost a year for the worst of the withdrawal symptoms to abate: night sweats, difficulty sleeping, headaches, hot flushes, a reduced sex drive and heart palpitations. It required daily forms of negotiation and it was difficult to constantly find myself disappointing my own expectations of what I felt I should have been capable of. Paige and I had this in common; the texture of her life changed dramatically during the induced menopause too. There was a sudden 'rigorous dailiness' in the change, as daily routines and rituals had to be altered to accommodate menopausal symptoms in us as young people, as young women. I cried constantly and for almost no reason; I was physically immobile because of the pain, and psychologically immobilised by sadness. For her, menopause 'kicked in pretty much overnight', just as my withdrawal symptoms did.

> I thought I was dying. I woke up drenched in sweat and I had the worst headache, and at first I thought I was having a heart attack or something. That continued pretty much the whole time, and I'd sit in the bath full of cold water frantically googling to confirm it was still just menopause.

Sex, sleeping and the shared spaces we inhabited with those we loved were perhaps the hardest to navigate; mediating between our altered experience of our bodies and what we wanted them to do.

So, I almost immediately just couldn't have sex.

I had the same experience; I went through a year and a half of being completely asexual. Sex became an unbearable discomfort.

I was PAINFULLY dry, and nothing could change that. It even seemed like my body was so dried up that it like soaked up lube, so sex was impossible for me. Which had a big toll on my relationship and my confidence, and also I am someone that just likes a lot of sex so I missed everything that comes with it. There's something very weird about not even being able to masturbate, it's one of those things you just take for granted.

I wanted to ask about the speed of it; how Paige was confronted with its immediacy, and its constancy; whether all the symptoms appeared at once or if it got worse over time?

The sweating and total vaginal dryness started straight away, and everything else within a month and got worse and worse over time.

I woke up at four o'clock every single morning like clockwork. I had night sweats and the most horrendous dreams. I headbutted my partner twice in the face! We laugh about it now, but it hurt too. It was another reminder that I had very little agency over the processes my body was enduring. I didn't know what was happening until it was happening. There was a relentlessness to our lives that it took time to adjust to.

The big thing for me was the flop sweats. I had to shower every single morning and completely strip the bed. We ended up having to throw the mattress away because it was so stained, even though we had three mattress protectors and I slept on a towel. It meant getting up earlier, etc., completely changing up my routine to be able to function. I am an evening shower person because that's when I go to the gym so I would shower there, but then have to shower again every morning because I'd be drenched through. A few times I woke up in the night and had to shower because I found it too gross to go back to sleep, and a few times I also slept in the bath because I was sick of having to change the sheets etc. I got a lot of UTIs [urinary tract infections] also which they told me is common but drove me up the wall, as I'd never even had thrush before.

Within an altered landscape of living Paige and I both held on to the little things, the small everyday things that made us feel like us; for me, I put all of myself into my coursework. In the time before I stopped taking the opiates, I was working on a final-year performance for my undergraduate drama degree. It was a physical theatre performance that considered exhaustion and failure. I dragged myself home from rehearsals feeling shattered and accomplished. During my MA, my poetic work became my life; it was what I found joy in. I wrote my entire dissertation in bed.

We found the things that made us feel like ourselves:

I found it really hard to carry on working out, but I still went to the gym every day because it was one of the few things that I had always done and could still do. So I wanted to hold on to something that was 'me', even though it hurt and was hell.

But it still hurt.

I was made constantly aware of which parts of my life I was displaying and which parts I was consciously making an effort to conceal, in order to make the rigours of this altered form of daily life invisible. I asked Paige if there were parts of induced menopause that she felt she had to hide from certain people, either because of their expected discomfort due to the 'taboo' of female healthcare, or because it was 'unprofessional', regardless of how noticeable the effects were. Paige's response was something that resonated profoundly:

All of it. I hid all of it. It was all gross and embarrassing, and men tend to react like you've just pooped on the floor if you dare to mention anything vaguely linked to a vagina/periods, etc. I work in a male-dominated industry, so I had to hide all of it.

In a political moment of strong, empowered and courageous female figures, I had often wondered if shame in itself was potential for shame. I hid my withdrawal symptoms as best I could and was often seen as somehow 'stronger' or more praiseworthy for trying to 'put on a brave face'.

I sometimes thought of make-up as warpaint, but I don't any more; I try to distance myself from a language of conflict and violence. I still, however, think of it as liquid confidence. Despite this, I think it was inevitable that some still grew irritable at visible signs of my discomfort. I became deeply uncomfortable with the way my body looked and felt, and that shame did become a source of embarrassment. I knew I had no reason to hide but I still wanted to; make-up and chest-binding consequently became substantially important, so that I could comport myself in a way that felt safe and that I could feel comfortable with.

There's a poem called 'Käthe Kollwitz' by Muriel Rukeyser that contains this stunning line in the third stanza – I think about it a lot in relation to the 'taboo' issue of women's healthcare:

> What would happen if one woman told the truth about
>   her life?
> The world would split   open

I find myself thinking about menopause as a 'world-splitting' event, in which the female body is 'split open', and about how we can respond to that truthfully and authentically, beginning with this truth: that we both found our bodies to be embarrassing.

> I felt like the sweating made me look like I was fat and out of shape, which
> I am sensitive about anyway. I felt like less of a woman because I couldn't
> even get myself off. I just didn't feel like a person any more.

I wanted to think critically about how disabling the symptoms of menopause can be for young people assigned female at birth, even as it's considered a form of 'treatment' for endometriosis. In considering menopause in relation to disability, I read Rosemarie Garland-Thomson's chapter, 'Disability, Identity, and Representation: An Introduction' from her book *Extraordinary Bodies*, in which she states: 'Disability is the attribution of corporeal deviance – not so much a property of bodies as a product of cultural rules about what bodies should be or do.'

The experience of menopause is not discrete – I do see disability and menopause as having an element of commonality and I was curious about Paige's opinion: did she think the experience of having an induced menopause as a young woman could be disabling? I was curious how much the stigma attached to that word – disability – would play into this, but to my surprise, she said: 'Yes'.

> Yes. It was also just very isolating. I couldn't hug anyone, couldn't hold a hand, couldn't even sit too near people. I had to keep away from everyone and it made me feel like everyone wanted to keep away from me.

I think it's also about what bodies should be *seen* to be or do. The 'world-splitting' is something of an inevitable experience for those assigned female at birth, and yet still considered taboo, unprofessional, or something to 'get over', like a sore throat or a bad day – despite its complete alteration of our day-to-day bodily experience – we're expected to carry on as normal. It perpetuates the idea that sickness is not to be seen. And yet in some regard, while choosing to undergo an induced menopause as a treatment is a refusal of bodily normalcy, it is also a choice; I wanted to know if that small amount of agency – knowing that technically she could stop it at any time – had an impact for Paige? She said that she had decided to stop: 'I wussed out'.

> I feel like I was forced into having it, and I don't think I'd understood how bad it would be. It was a bit like they'd tried everything else, so I was browbeaten into trying the last option. The doctors wanted me to keep going, but I genuinely thought I was going to kill myself. I couldn't do it. It might have gotten better in time, but I was so alone and so sad all the time. They pushed me quite hard to stick at it, which is when I got the anti-depressants as well, but I couldn't do it.

I think undergoing a medically induced menopause can certainly be seen as an event in which the female body is 'split open', as it becomes enmeshed within a system of healthcare and of capitalism, and entangled with multitudinous and often competing systems. It can feel at times like your own body is not entirely your own. I was curious what this meant for care, particularly self-care, and what it was like when it felt like the body was not your own to take care of or look after?

> I don't get to make any decisions about anything, not really. They are all too afraid of me suing one day or things like this. The system is made to

be risk averse and that means that you get steamrollered into a one-size-fits-all treatment. But that treatment didn't work for me. At the moment they are trying to force me to either try menopause again or have the same invasive surgery I HAVE ALREADY HAD THAT DIDN'T WORK again. They won't do what I want unless I have another child, but I am not financially ready to have another child.

The pressure to be a 'good' patient, one that conforms to treatment and doesn't become 'troublesome', can be stifling and, at times, overwhelming. It stopped me from asking more of my GP, about what side-effects might occur, and what could happen to my body. By the time I started asking, they didn't know the answers. I asked if Paige had the same experience – whether she was given flyers, or told to look at the NHS website?

LOTS of flyers, and websites, and encouraged to go to a support group that was over an hour away. I think because they were so desperate for me to try it, they glossed over the symptoms. There was a lot of focus from my GP (who is also my mother's GP) on how easy my family had found menopause and so it would be easy for me.

When systems of care fail or come up short, I think this is when the act of self-care becomes most important. I was asked repeatedly to keep a pain journal by my GP, and I inquired if Paige was ever asked to track her menopause on a micro level, not just a macro one of perseverance and struggle.

I had an app to track my bleeding and my pain to see if it was working as a treatment for my endo.

Within illness and moments of physical change, I became aware of just how communal the body becomes as it is processed through not just the NHS system, but language, lovers, friends, family, doctors, nurses, apps and the wider societal discourse. Each of these offers forms of advice when a body acts in what is perceived to be an abnormal fashion and at times it can be hard to know who to trust, or at least who to listen and be attentive to. In this regard, my friends have been an astounding source of support and solidarity; our horror stories sound the same.

I saw three different doctors because the first two offended me. The first two were men, and I dislike being told to 'just get on with it', etc. by someone who literally doesn't even have the organs they are talking about so has no idea what it is actually like. The third was a woman, and her I liked and trusted. That doesn't mean I didn't still Google everything, because I did, but I trusted her as much as you can trust anyone when it comes to things as sensitive as your health and body.

It would be difficult to see this as utterly disconnected from the crisis that frequently describes the NHS; chronically underfunded and short-staffed, we know navigating this collapsing entity is only made more difficult by the fact we are female, by the fact we are young and, for me, the fact I am non-white and gender non-conforming.

At the moment the issue with austerity is that they've been stupid and cut vasectomies – they are no longer on the NHS in my county. They're looking at changing it, but this means that if I want to have sex, I have to handle the contraception as they will not give my husband a vasectomy. All contraception messes with either my endo or my drugs. It's absolutely driving me mad.

Also, the most recent specialist I saw openly refused to do anything until I have a second child and kept insisting that as I'd married so young my second husband would want a baby. He put the fictional desires of some fictional 'second husband' (again, as far as he knows I am happily married to my first and only husband) above my need to be healthy and function and take care of my daughter. He's lucky he still has all his teeth, to be honest.

As a result, I'm interested in the voices we do pay attention to. Which women's voices have I listened to the most? Perhaps unsurprisingly, most of the people I've turned to for advice have been the online disability communities that are comprised primarily of advocates and those living with disability rather than 'medical professionals'.

Facebook groups of other people taking the same treatment, etc., and a lady I met in the hospital when having the shots – we became quite good friends.

To what extent had my mother's experiences influenced my expectations and perceptions of menopause? I became curious how the women around us shape our predictions of our own bodies, and discovered that I was not alone in feeling this influence:

> Both my grandmother and my mother had very late and incredibly easy menopause. It is because of how easy they both found it that I agreed to have it induced, as I essentially thought that as they could do it, I could too. I did not understand how different it would be. I am still sort of hoping that I will end up having 'real' menopause late and easy, but it is doubtful I'll make it much longer before I have a hysterectomy anyway.

It was after talking to Paige that I knew, regardless of my diagnosis, that I would never have an induced menopause. In her concise words: 'In all honesty, I don't think it's worth it.' But I know there's a likely chance that I still may go through it someday and, in truth, that scares me too. The women in my family are ill; all the women in my mother's family are ill. When I became sick at 19, I suddenly had more in common with my mother, with my aunt, with my great-aunt and with my baby first cousin than I ever had before. It felt like an inheritance. We suddenly shared this medical language of long diagnostic names, drug names and chronic precarity.

Reaching the critical age

When I was unable to sleep due to the pain, I would sometimes get out of bed and make my way to the kitchen to make myself a cup of tea, always English Breakfast. Walking down the hallway, if I saw the living-room lights on through the glass in the doors it meant that my mother was up too – kept awake by the menopausal hot flushes that worsened the insomnia she's had for almost thirty years. As her first menopause symptoms began when I was four, it intimidates me to think that her symptoms have lasted almost as long as my lifetime. But I am a little hopeful that things will change; when I asked her about what menopause was first like she said:

I was quite happy about this initially, after having painful monthly periods for twenty-five years and then almost painless periods for another fifteen, due to the birth of my only child.

She was never able to take contraceptives for the pain that her periods caused, and thankfully I have. I do dare to be a tiny bit hopeful here; perhaps things will have changed so that by the time I am 'old' the menopause I experience won't impact the disabled body I have quite so severely.

As someone who is young and queer, I have been thinking about menopause in relation to pride: to queer pride, to crip pride, and whether there is a possibility for a form of menopausal pride? To be proud in the fact that it's something experienced or experiencing – a type of 'menopride' perhaps? Suffice to say I think the idea horrified my mother a little.

No! There is nothing great about reaching a certain age when everything starts declining and deteriorating!!

She even used two exclamation marks, so I knew she wasn't joking. There are thirty-seven years between us, and I do feel them pronouncedly around discussions like this one. We'd never talked about menopause before I came to write this, even if we talk about chronic illness almost constantly. My mother sees it as an almost exclusively melancholy process:

Since menopause is usually connected with the ageing process later in life, it has a huge negative impact, leading to some grief with a letting go of youth and fertility, an 'unwelcome stranger' and 'intruder' who never goes away, but deepens its hold on the body, weaving its effect to every cell, every pore ... weakening, ageing, destroying life and vitality.

I hope my experience will be a different one. My life changed drastically when I became disabled, and it's changed drastically again recently in leaving the UK and returning to Singapore to undertake a PhD. I hope I will not mourn change; I hope I will instead appreciate the new and unexpected little things that I discover along the way.

I'm looking forward to trying what Paige calls 'happy bread' when I'm older; it's bread infused with CBD (cannabidiol, a non-psychoactive chemical from the *Cannabis sativa* plant used for pain management), that she buys from her local bakery, and which she says is delicious! Maybe I will appreciate going for long walks in winter, or the ever-present air-conditioning in Singapore. I look forward to the day when my body is no longer a surprise, when I am older and doctors believe me when I tell them I am sick, and treat me in a way that is entirely un-fussy.

I hope one day that if I have to be menopausal, that I will be menopausal and proud.

Note on chapter
Quote from Lisa Robertson's *Proverbs of a She-Dandy* used by permission of the author. Fragment from 'Käthe Kollwitz' © Muriel Rukeyser used by permission of the author. Quote from Rosemarie Garland-Thomson's chapter, 'Disability, Identity, and Representation: An Introduction', from her book *Extraordinary Bodies* used by permission of the author.

Cat Chong is a poet, a recent graduate of the Poetic Practice MA at Royal Holloway, and a current PhD student at Nanyang Technological University (NTU) in Singapore. Their work explores connections between stories of sickness in female-authored Singaporean and South East Asian illness narratives to investigate how intersections between gender and medicine have affected contemporary perceptions of illness. Their poetry has been featured in *Ache* magazine, Bad Betty Press's *Alter Egos* anthology, *Stride* online magazine and in the Crested Tit Collective anthology *Harpies*. They are non-binary and also a co-founder of the Crested Tit Collective. Their work has been performed at the Theatre of Failure, shown at the Small Publishers Fair and can be found in the National Poetry Library, the BookArtBookshop and Senate House Library. Their interests include ecology, feminism, contemporary poetics, medical humanities and disability studies.

12

Men O Pause

Acclaimed graphic artist and Fine Art lecturer Emily Steinberg visualises the history of menopause and what it has meant to her.

For over a thousand years, menopause has been treated as an illness, something to be feared and fixed. *Men O Pause*, my graphic narrative presented here, focuses on the grim and creepy history of how menopausal women have been misperceived, mistreated, operated on and even murdered because of their age and lack of ovarian function. In 2020, not only do we no longer need to be 'fixed', but we are quite happy to be living outside the realm of women's historical natural function.

Note on chapter
Information researched from 'Mad with Menopause: The way we look at The Change has certainly, well, changed', by Jackie Rosenhek, *Doctor's Review*, February 2014.

MEN O PAUSE

THE IDEA of MENOPAUSE, of BLEEDING AND NOT BLEEDING, SO MYSTERIOUS, SO of WOMAN...

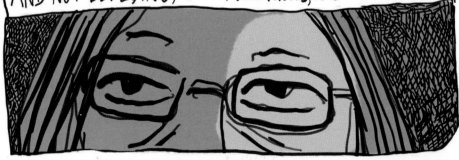

IS TIED UP IN THE NOTION THAT A WOMAN WHO IS DRIED UP, HER WOMB DEAD, IS NO LONGER USEFUL.

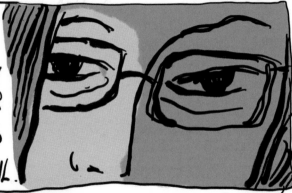

THEN, BECAUSE SHE IS NO LONGER USEFUL SHE BECOMES DANGEROUS...

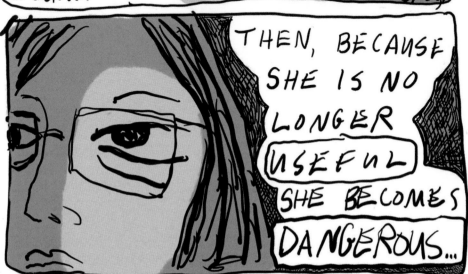

(1)

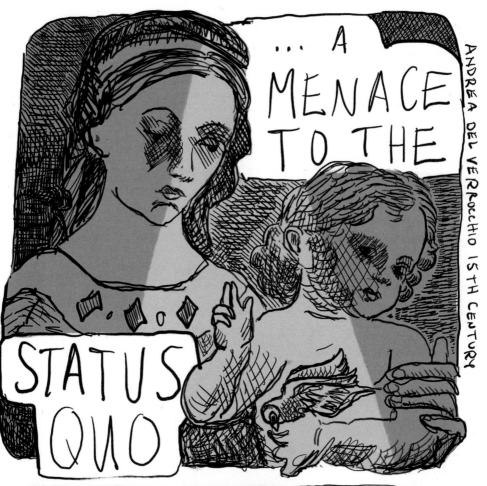

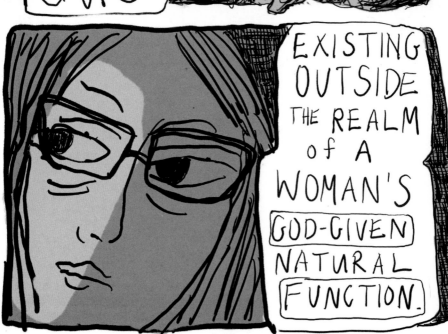

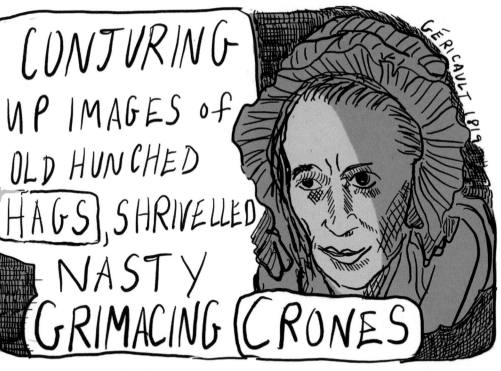

CONJURING UP IMAGES of OLD HUNCHED HAGS, SHRIVELLED NASTY GRIMACING CRONES

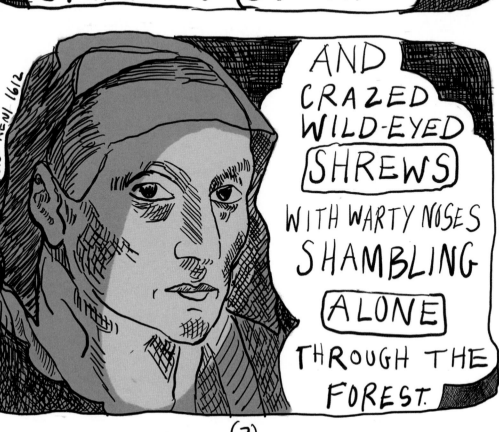

AND CRAZED WILD-EYED SHREWS WITH WARTY NOSES SHAMBLING ALONE THROUGH THE FOREST.

(3)

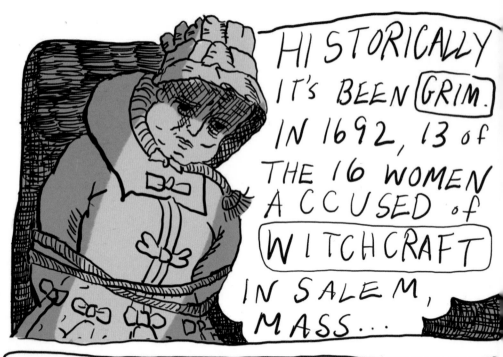

HISTORICALLY IT'S BEEN GRIM. IN 1692, 13 of THE 16 WOMEN ACCUSED of WITCHCRAFT IN SALEM, MASS...

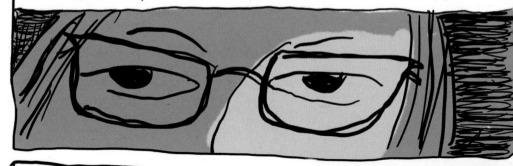

WERE PAST CHILD-BEARING AGE...

AND PERCEIVED AS POWERFUL THREATENING AND UNGODLY

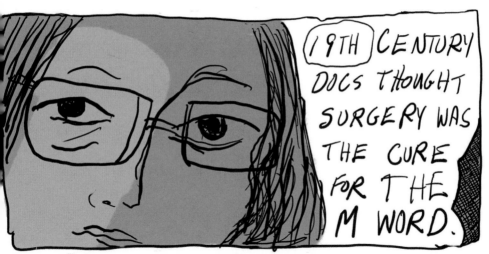

19TH CENTURY DOCS THOUGHT SURGERY WAS THE CURE FOR THE M WORD.

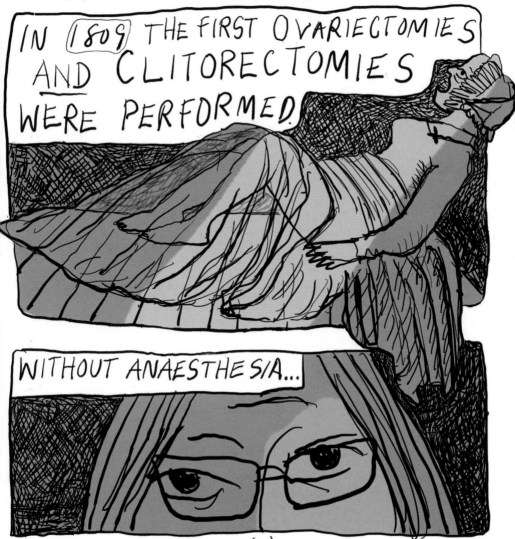

IN 1809 THE FIRST OVARIECTOMIES AND CLITORECTOMIES WERE PERFORMED.

WITHOUT ANAESTHESIA...

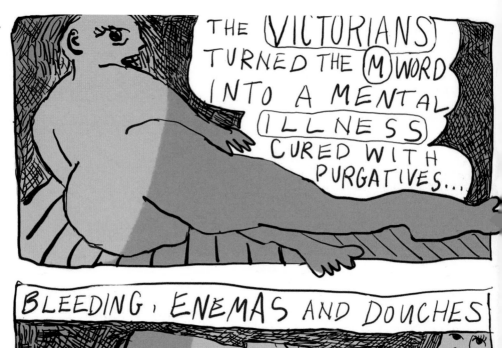

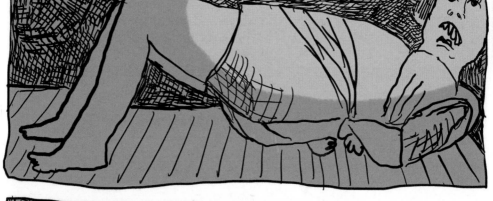

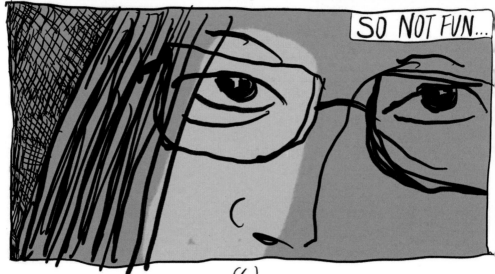

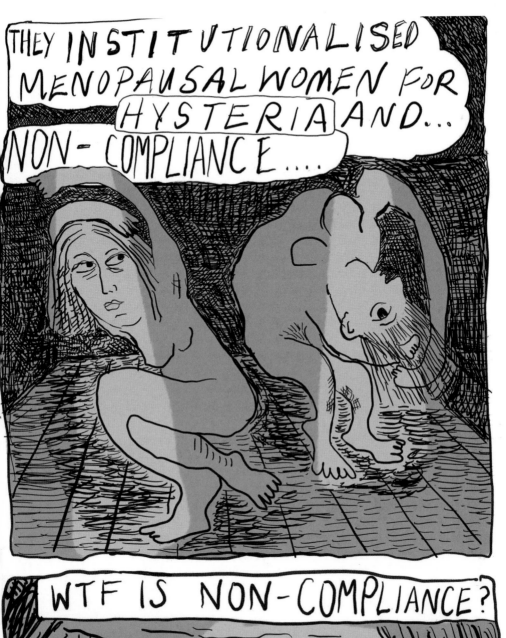

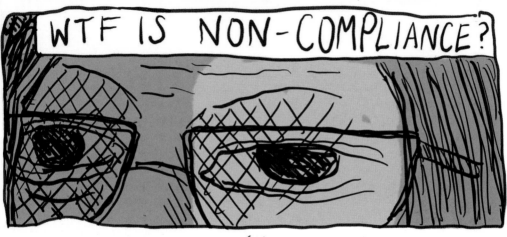

IN THE MID 20TH CENTURY, POLITE SOCIETY REMAINED LARGELY SILENT ON THE MATTER PEOPLE DIDN'T TALK ABOUT IT.

IT WAS JUST THAT THING THAT HAPPENED TO OLDER WOMEN... AND WHO CARED ANYWAY?

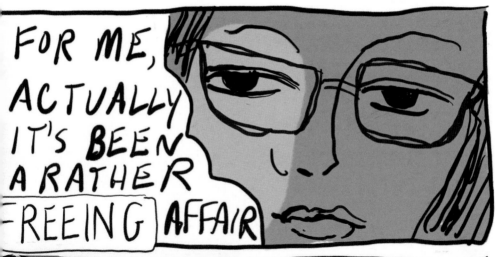

FOR ME, ACTUALLY IT'S BEEN A RATHER FREEING AFFAIR

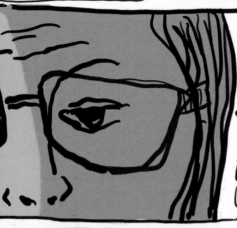

IT CAME ON EARLY WHICH SUCKED AS I WANTED CHILDREN. BUT THAT'S A WHOLE OTHER STORY....

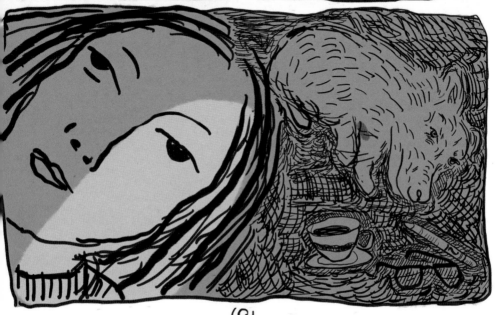

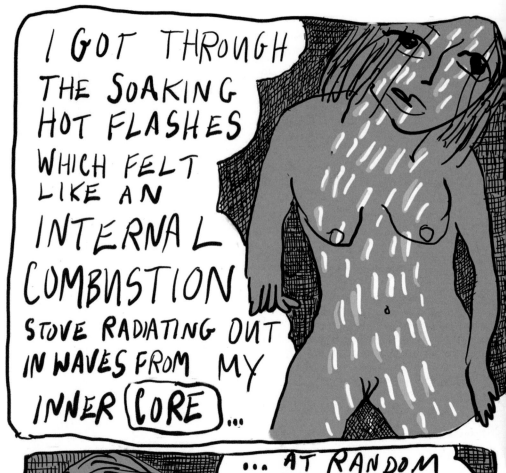

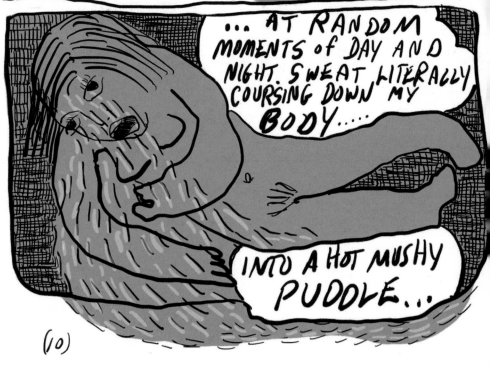

(10)

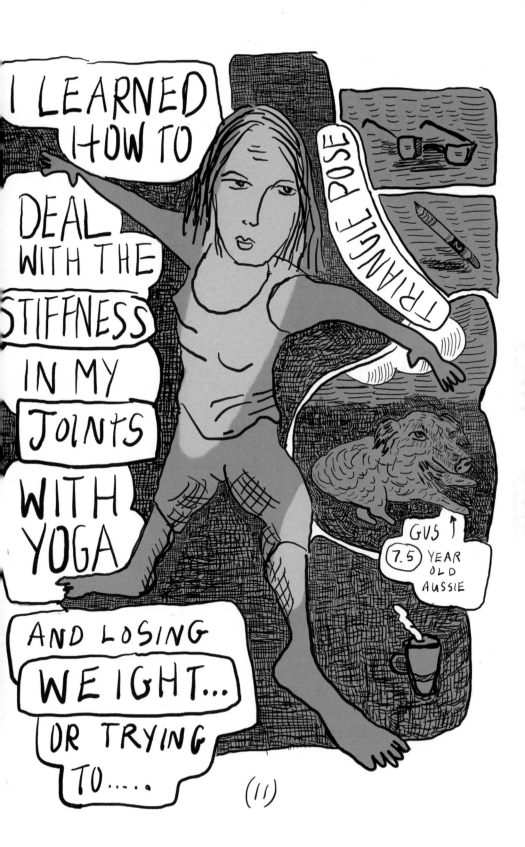

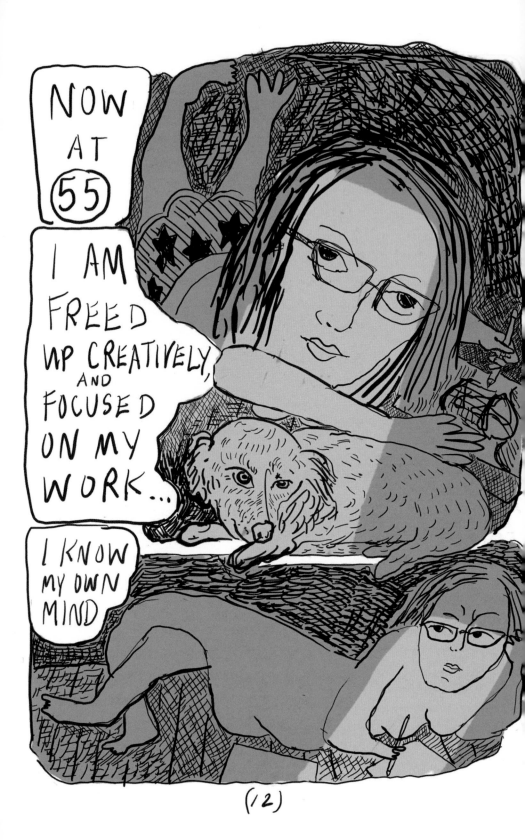

NOW AT (55)

I AM FREED UP CREATIVELY, AND FOCUSED ON MY WORK...

I KNOW MY OWN MIND

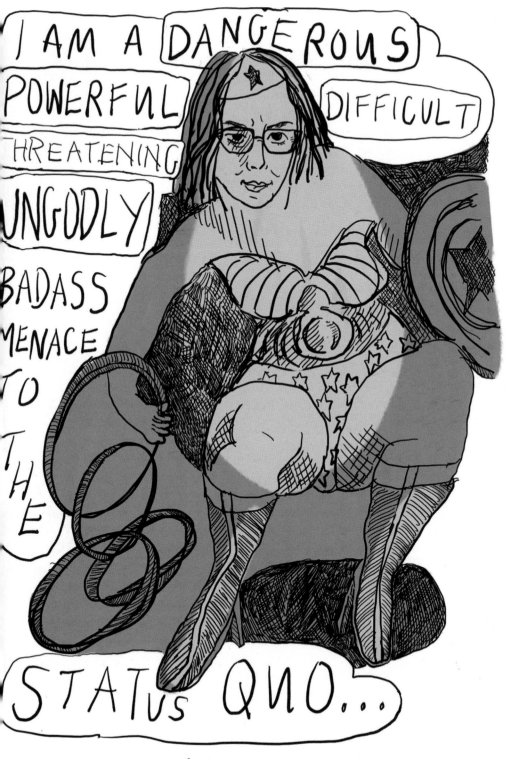

(13)

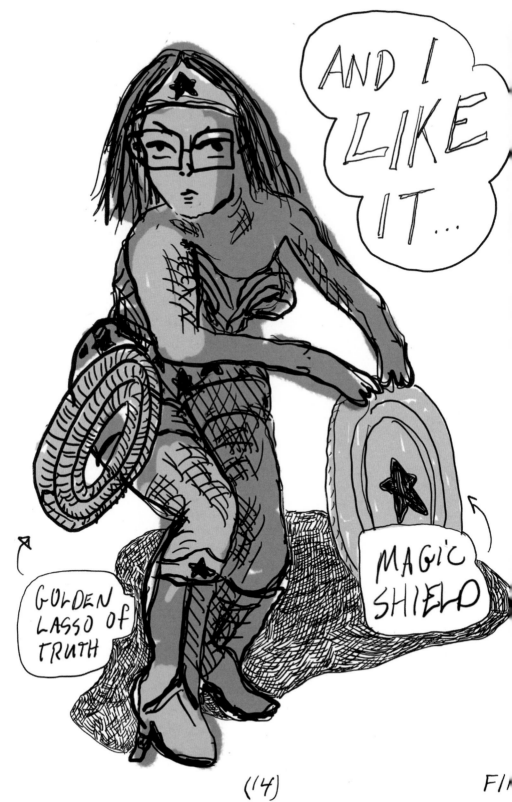

Emily Steinberg is an American artist, writer and educator whose work has been shown across the US and Europe. Most recently, her first cartoon was accepted into *The New Yorker* magazine and will be published in 2020. She has been named the first Artist in Residence at Drexel College of Medicine in Philadelphia, where she works with medical students to translate their medical school experiences into words and images. Her visual narratives have been regularly published in *Cleaver* magazine since 2013 and since summer 2019 she has taken on the role of visual narrative editor at *Cleaver*. Her memoir, *Graphic Therapy*, was published serially in *Smith* magazine and her short comic *Blogging Towards Oblivion* was included in *The Moment* (HarperCollins). She is a lecturer in Fine Art at Penn State University, Abington College, where she has been teaching since 2011. Steinberg earned her Master of Fine Arts from the University of Pennsylvania in Philadelphia.

13

Making the M-Word Go Viral

Aisling Grimley, founder of the hugely successful online community My Second Spring, and Ireland's first menopause coach **Catherine O'Keeffe** (aka Wellness Warrior.ie) explore the mystery of perimenopause and the power of sharing our experiences and knowledge.

Aisling Grimley

I've been lucky enough in that none of my symptoms were as incapacitating as they can be for some women. But still, I found perimenopause unsettling. I had mood swings, rage, breast tenderness, irregular periods, which were disruptive enough to send me looking for answers. At first it didn't dawn on me that this might be anything to do with menopause – why should it? I was young, and no one in my peer group was talking about menopause. Like many women, I thought I might be pregnant, until a pregnancy test confirmed that I wasn't.

This was 2013, a time when no one said the word 'menopause' out loud, even at a book club – and perimenopause was a term rarely encountered outside medical websites. To be honest, it was something I'd not given the slightest thought to. As someone who has always tried to be well informed and proactive about general health, this was a first for me. When I mentioned menopause to friends, most knew nothing, and those who did had negative associations. Menopause was for other, much older, women. It connoted decline and deterioration and invisibility. It seemed crazy to me then that a physical change experienced by 100 per cent of women should be so shrouded in silence and shame.

As well as wanting answers for myself, I also wanted to tackle this taboo. Having four daughters, mine is a house full of girls, and I didn't want to pass on this sense of darkness around what is a natural female life stage, so I decided to be open about menopause.

I started to research menopause online and was amazed to find no local resource and very little relatable information. So, I set up My Second Spring in 2013, following a digital media course that I did at the European Communications Institute in Dublin and literally from my kitchen table. The idea was to provide information and inspiration, and bring a new and more upbeat perspective to menopause as a time of new beginnings – the 'second spring' that is revered in Chinese culture, where menopause is viewed much more positively. I wanted to give women like myself somewhere they could go to access good-quality information about menopause, but more importantly where they might find a sense of community – and the reassurance that they were not on their own. One of the biggest issues with menopause being taboo for so long is that women don't feel comfortable admitting to others that they are in menopause. The label has such negative associations, you can understand why women are in no hurry to assume it. So, women don't talk. They don't admit to the night sweats that rob them of their sleep, the vaginal atrophy and urinary tract infections that can steal their sex lives and their relationships, the debilitating fatigue that can make getting through the working day so much more challenging. They don't perhaps realise that the thinning hair, the accelerated skin ageing and the weight gain could be a result of their changing hormones and that there is so much help if they know where to look. They might be having crippling psychological symptoms of anxiety, anger, mood swings, paranoia, low mood, insomnia, but don't realise why, just that they feel dreadful. They honestly can feel like they are going mad. And not talking makes it ten times worse.

Knowing that really spurred me on to make a change.

At first, the site had a small local following. I really nudged my comfort zone in holding events for women reaching menopause and talking about the subject on TV and radio, mainly in Ireland. At the time, it felt like I was the only woman openly talking menopause on-screen, and I became something of a 'go-to' person for commentary on women's experience at midlife – not what I had originally envisioned in my career path!

Very quickly it became clear that women wanted to read about and hear about menopause. The audience grew to around 8,000 visitors daily within three years. Women shared their issues and symptoms on the site, and I realised that this was indeed a resource that was long overdue.

Who visits My Second Spring?

The audience for My Second Spring is millions of women from all five continents, but mostly in Ireland and the UK. We have women visitors ranging in age from 30 to 70, and some men, too, but mainly it is women in their late forties and early fifties who are in the throes of a tough menopause and desperately want some direction. We have had women writing to us seeking advice for their teenage daughters, who are going through the heartbreak of an early menopause, or what is termed 'premature ovarian insufficiency' (POI). We have stories from women in their seventies who are in constant discomfort from vaginal atrophy, and women who feel so distressed by their basket of symptoms that they have ended up leaving their jobs.

It has been stunning to connect with women all over the world from my laptop in the kitchen and to realise how much we all share. On a daily basis I get messages from women in Australia, New Zealand, the US and the UK saying they are so glad to find us and realise they aren't alone and that they aren't going crazy. That's been the most rewarding and the most motivating part of the My Second Spring story. This extract, from an email I received from Lina, in Indonesia, is an example of the kinds of feedback I have received:

Hi Aisling,
My name is Lina. I'll be 50 soon in April. I am a mom of one son aged 13. I am from Yogyakarta, Indonesia ... I was very happy when I found your website just at the end of 2019. It is great & really a big help for me.

I had my last period in May 2018 when I was 48. I am postmenopausal but I still have some symptoms ... In fact, I didn't have severe symptoms in the years prior to it. I only had missed periods, hair loss & brittle nails ... But soon after that at the end of July 2018 I started to get terrible ones – dizziness, insomnia, night sweat, fatigue, brain fog, depression, anxiety and many more. Until then I didn't know that they were related to menopause. It was my elder sister who told me ...

There's a lot of information about menopause on the internet in Indonesian ... But it seems it was not written by those who really experienced it. They give tips to make it smooth. But those tips aren't as easy & simple as they say. For me, they are only theoretical writings. They do not tell how it feels to be menopausal. Personal stories from women who have experienced menopause in Indonesian are very rare ...

Unable to find info about menopause first hand from the women who experienced it, I started to browse in English ... The true stories from women somewhere very far from my country – on the other side of the world – relieved my stress. What made me surprised was that some of them had exactly the same feelings I got – initially, I thought I was severely ill and would die soon; and also I was afraid I was going crazy because I felt my head was full of weird things. OMG...

The stories and the comments from other women on your website meant a lot to me. They were a relief ... previously I had believed that I must have been the most unfortunate, the unluckiest one because I had suffered a lot while other women hadn't – while in fact it was all because I never talked about menopause with anyone & also nobody ever told me about it before, even my late mom. And I never knew or saw someone, a woman around me, suffering from menopause symptoms like me. Never... My elder sister knew it but she had never told me until I experienced it. Just like in other parts of the world, it is considered as a taboo.

I really love your website, Aisling. Thank you very much for creating such a great one. Thank you for sharing.

Our most-visited pages are those that answer the most common problems women first notice in midlife, the ones that really worry them: fatigue, low mood, anxiety, insomnia, missed periods. Strangely, hot flushes, the commonest but probably most benign of menopause symptoms, are not top of the list.

We take the approach of a best friend, and the site speaks to women in that friendly, conversational tone – it complements the more formal style of medical sites, and women tell us they appreciate it. The open-forum nature of the comments section also allows women to swap experiences, symptoms, solutions, advice and tips – and that is a very valuable resource; the wisdom of women never fails to impress me.

The sense of being 'one of many' in menopause is a real comfort; it takes away the isolation. Some of the women who write to me have heartbreaking stories to tell. They are at a time of life when bereavement, caring for frail parents, caring for children, demanding jobs, relationship difficulties could all be part of the mix and then – wham, nature delivers menopause with its reputed forty or more symptoms. It is not difficult to see why suicide rates in women, while considerably lower than those for men of the same age, are at their highest between 45 and 54 in both the Republic of Ireland and UK, as reported in The Samaritans' 'Suicide Statistics Report' in December 2019. While My Second Spring focuses on the hope and positivity of being a woman in your fifties, we have to meet women where they are: overloaded, stretched too thin, stressed out and floored by symptoms as some are.

Finally, we cover solutions for menopause symptoms for those women for whom hormone replacement therapy (HRT) is not an option – some women are in recovery from breast cancer, others feel strongly about avoiding HRT. Changes in lifestyle habits can make an enormous difference to a woman's experience of menopause, whether or not she opts for hormonal therapy. Adopting good exercise, nutrition, sleep and stress-management habits can lessen the severity of symptoms like hot flushes, night sweats and weight gain, and will help sustain women through the second half of their lives.

In 2020, Ireland is in a very positive place in terms of the menopause conversation. The Irish media have been supportive over the last five years, discussing the subject in an intelligent, non-sensational way, which has helped hugely in breaking open the taboo. The impact of celebrities in the UK and beyond 'coming out' about their experience of menopause has been significant, and while as yet we have no prominent Irish media stars making headlines about menopause, there are now regular interviews with women in the media, and menopause-themed events happening every week around Ireland.

Anna Mooney, Catherine O'Keeffe and I thought about putting on a conference for women in menopause a few years ago, as the only menopause event at the time was the Irish Menopause Society's annual conference, which was not open to women outside the medical and healthcare professions. That situation seemed absurd to me – that valuable information about this taboo subject affecting half the population at midlife would be so off-bounds to the very women who were going through menopause. So I started small, with a regular series of 'Meet the Experts' events in Dublin, covering topics ranging from sex at menopause, to exercise and nutrition, to changing up your second act. Then, as menopause moved into the mainstream in 2019, we decided it was time to assemble all of our menopause experts and specialists in one venue for a full day of information and inspiration for women: The M Word event. At our next event we plan to tackle vaginal and sexual health; nutrition; options for HRT; what to do if you can't or don't want to take HRT; skincare at midlife and a wide range of other topics.

When women have knowledge, they are empowered to make good decisions for their well-being. The My Second Spring website and events can go so far, but we need menopause awareness and conversations to reach every corner of society.

It has been incredible to watch global awareness of menopause grow exponentially since I started My Second Spring in October 2013. At that time, I felt like a crazy maverick and people asked me why I had chosen to be the 'poster girl' for such an unpopular topic. Maybe it was my past career in PR that made me feel the image of menopause needed a makeover. I certainly believed then as now that women needed to own the topic and help younger women to get support rather than feeling isolated. No longer should menopause be for other women, it should be for every woman.

Catherine O'Keeffe

Hindsight is great, especially when it comes to perimenopause. Looking back, I didn't recognise at the time the subtle changes that were occurring – it was only when I stopped, took time and looked at my body and life as a whole that I realised I was actually in perimenopause at the age of 44. My life underwent a complete change at this stage. I was restless in my job, and I was looking for another adventure in my life ... something new. Twinned with this were those subtle signs of perimenopause: my periods changed in terms of flow and became heavier; premenstrual symptoms that I hadn't had in years, like breast tenderness, bloating and mood swings, came back. It all happened very gradually and still today my changes are slow and gradual. Throughout my life I have developed skills which have been invaluable in handling perimenopause, and I have been lucky that my symptoms have been manageable so far. Now, aged 50, my periods are totally erratic and come like intermittent celebrations.

While I have been fortunate in my journey through perimenopause to date, I see first hand those women who suffer more harshly through this transition. I grew up with complementary medicine – my mum gave me a great foundation in it – and I work with many women who can navigate menopause with complementary medicine and lifestyle tweaks, but there are women who may need hormone replacement therapy (HRT) and require medical treatment to live a normal life through the menopause. We only get one life and I believe we have to live it to the max, and that should not include suffering needlessly. Menopause differs for every woman on the planet, and it makes sense that treatment options will differ to meet those needs. As Iris Murdoch said, 'There is no typical menopause, there are as many menopauses as women' (*The Good Apprentice*, 1985). For me, the important part is that women are aware of the choices – empowerment comes from knowing you have options.

Daily, here in Ireland, I see that women do not know about the options available to them – whether it is complementary or HRT. If you Google 'menopause', the results are staggering, and for any women experiencing brain fog, anxiety and concentration issues, navigating the information and the options is daunting. This is where we need to see change: women need the key factual information so they can make empowering, informed personal choices.

As I entered perimenopause, I began to realise that I wanted a change of direction in my life and, having previously studied complementary medicine, working in women's health was a natural route. I also saw the need for more information about menopause – the knowledge simply was not there. Aisling had previously set up My Second Spring, which became a great resource for women not just in Ireland but globally – you can see there how women support each other on a daily basis. I began writing blogs for the site and then established Wellness Warrior, an independent menopause service, sharing knowledge, bringing menopause to the workplace, working one-on-one with women and also 'taking to the road': travelling around Ireland talking with and supporting women to understand what menopause really is about. It's not just the hot flushes and the night sweats – it is so much more. Those symptoms are just the tip of the iceberg; underneath there can be anxiety, depression, vaginal atrophy, brain fog, bladder issues, loss of confidence, exhaustion and so on. Libido sexual health, vaginal atrophy, pelvic core health and depression are key areas that need more open discussion and support.

When my mum was going through menopause, while I was growing up, it was never discussed. Did she ever chat to her friends or family about it? I don't think so. Now aged 90 and with dementia, she can't give me those answers, but it was certainly an era of 'grin and bear it'. I remember getting my periods (certainly the same time my mum was peak menopause) and there was no discussion, only a *Girls Talk* book slipped under my pillow. How things have changed on that front – and this gives me hope for menopause. My mum has a great sense of humour, and had menopause been openly discussed I think we could as a family have supported her more and even laughed through parts of it. Like those Sunday roast dinners when she looked hotter than if she had stepped out of a sauna! Talking, sharing, education, treatment options can all help make the journey through menopause easier. After all, menopause is a family journey, impacting all relationships.

As everyone's experience of menopause is different, each woman needs to explore treatment methods and see what she finds beneficial. I believe the choices women have come down to three alternatives: complementary therapies, HRT, or a blend of both – there is simply no one size that fits all. If you are using complementary therapies, you still need to make lifestyle adjustments like exercise and nutrition, and the same applies if you opt for HRT. A blended approach sees women using HRT alongside complementary therapies like acupuncture, herbalism, reflexology, homeopathy and so on, all supported by optimum lifestyle choices. Being prepared going into perimenopause can make this transition easier – that means starting in your early forties (for natural menopause). Embracing these well-known lifestyle habits – food, movement, sleep, stress, brain health – that will provide a strong foundation for your health in menopause.

Women also need a trusted and supportive GP. In Ireland, we are moving forward but we have a long way to go. Take, for example, HRT. Many women are not informed of the various forms of HRT, and often they are not told about the possibilities available. When you make a visit to your GP, you should be able to feel confident in the knowledge that menopause was a key part of their formal training and not an add-on after completion. Across Ireland we are seeing more and more GPs enhancing their knowledge of menopause, which is a great step forward, but it needs to be introduced in medical training and become a bigger part of the overall medical picture.

As a menopause coach, working with women in Ireland and all over the world, my goal is to empower each woman with the knowledge and tools to help her deal with symptoms as they come up – a personal toolkit. This normally covers specific symptom management, nutrition, exercise, self-care and general lifestyle habits. I am lucky to have a wealth of experience and knowledge to work with and share, and my passion is to help as many women as possible. This is the benefit of bringing women together, as happens when I do a Perimenopause Unplugged event. This is a public event where I talk about menopause in detail, covering all aspects from symptoms and treatment options to lifestyle. I can reach more women in one sitting and therefore can help more women. The same applies to The M Word (Ireland's first menopause summit), which I co-founded with Aisling and Anna Mooney from Omnia Media. This is a great gathering for women to explore and discuss life and menopause.

My background in the corporate world gave me the opportunity to work with people from different countries and diverse backgrounds. It was a challenging job – in both the positive and more difficult sense. I learned a great deal, and I met some amazing people: managing a large team over multiple global locations certainly has its challenges. Women generally tend to be hard on themselves and this is very evident in the corporate world, where you are continually striving to maintain your place and your reputation. We feel we have more to prove. The next generation will hopefully approach this differently but, certainly, women push themselves hard. The multitasking of home life, family, ageing parents, relationships and work are tricky to balance and even more so in menopause. The 'caregiver burden' is an added complexity to menopause.

While the corporate world has changed over recent years, and these changes have been for the better – more women in senior roles, moves towards gender equality in pay, flexible working hours – there is still a long way to go, and still a gap in menopause support. A crucial step forward will see menopause as a leadership discussion embraced by executive-level managers and the implementation of menopause-supporting policies in companies and workplaces. The catalyst here is women managers support-ing menopause. Women are working longer: that is a fact. Employers need to appreciate this and value the knowledge and experience older women bring to the workplace. A number of other cultures around the world dis-play a higher regard for women as they reach menopause, where they are respected for the vast wisdom they have gathered over the years – is it not an utter shame if we do not respect and value this too?

Women want to learn about menopause – they are starved of knowledge! They want to talk and share their stories. Nothing makes me smile more than doing a talk and seeing women who don't know each other sharing their experiences and nodding in agreement and support. When women support each other something magical happens. I often see women leav-ing a talk looking lighter as they realise what they are going through is normal – they aren't mad! Brain fog, fear of dementia, is very real at this time, and keeping our brains nourished is an integral part of your lifestyle plan and future-proofing your brain for the years ahead. *The XX Brain* by Dr Lisa Mosconi is an invaluable resource here. We can also be slow to discuss the impact of anxiety and depression in menopause, and once we open the conversation it helps women move forward. And they leave with a plan: understanding symptoms more and understanding where they can go for help and support.

My passion is for women to know their choices, to know the facts – plain and simple. That means understanding HRT, the benefits and the risks (based on factual evidence-based information, not media sensationalism), understanding complementary therapies and the essential lifestyle tweaks that have to be made. In Ireland, for example, many women have gotten into the habit of the nightly glass of wine – I am seeing this more and more – but the risks associated with alcohol and its impact on women's health are greatly understated. The British Menopause Society has drawn attention to the increased risk of breast cancer, for example. For every 1,000 women aged 50 to 59, research suggests twenty-three will go on to develop breast cancer in the next five years, but among women drinking two or more units of alcohol a day the figure is twenty-eight in 1,000. We would do Irish women (and women globally) a great justice if we launched a national campaign highlighting the long-term effects of alcohol. Recently, I spoke to a woman who was suffering severe night sweats. She was using an oestrogen patch, and while other symptoms had improved, this had not – as a nightly wine drinker it was not going to improve without addressing her alcohol intake. So, while we need to educate women more on all the treatment options, we also need more education on the various 'nutrient robbers', as I call them: alcohol, smoking, sugar, caffeine, stress. All in moderation.

Another layer of menopause education is reaching minority groups and ensuring all women in society have access to the support and information they need. The challenges faced by women from minority groups can be incredibly difficult, and there are inherent obstacles within specific groups, along with a lack of education and support. Many women in Ireland are working extremely hard at grassroots level to change this, but there is a long road ahead of us. The Irish Health Service Executive recently opened the doors to talking about menopause with the Travelling Community and its representatives – this group within Ireland has had very little access or exposure to menopause education. I was thrilled to be part of this exercise and welcome all opportunities to speak to as many women – and men – from different sectors of society as possible. We need to make sure that all those who might benefit are supported, including, for example, those with intellectual disabilities, Down's syndrome, conditions such as multiple sclerosis (MS), and women in prison. We need a centralised pool of knowledge that, like an octopus, can reach out to all parts of society.

In essence, this needs to be a global initiative where all countries finally address menopause for the inevitable life change it is. I have three sons and they are now as familiar with menopause and all it entails, as they are with pregnancy. This needs to be part of education at all levels: schools, healthcare providers and workplaces.

Inspired by Diane Danzebrink's brilliant and effective campaign, #MakeMenopauseMatter, and having met Diane in 2019, this campaign is the basis of the #MakeMenopauseMatterIreland initiative, which was launched by Diane at The M Word in October 2019. #MakeMenopauseMatterIreland is supported by Uplift, Ireland's largest campaigning community, connecting people to take action for a better Ireland.

We have four key objectives:

Menopause in the healthcare system: We want to see education for all women and families, and same-sex relationships. Education for minority groups – for example, women with intellectual disabilities and the Travelling Community. Education around the choices women have –

lifestyle, medical, etc. Enhanced education and awareness for GPs in relation to menopause – far too many women are suffering as GPs receive very little, if any, menopause education during their training, leaving them ill equipped to recognise and manage a phase of life that will directly affect at least 50 per cent of the population.

Menopause in the workplace: To raise awareness within the workplace and for all employers to have menopause guidelines in place to be able to support women experiencing symptoms. Too many women feel unsupported at work and currently one in ten leave the workplace due to menopause symptoms.

Secondary-school education: To introduce menopause education into the Personal, Social and Health Education (PSHE) curriculum for all teenage boys and girls. Every woman and man deserves to understand this phase of life. Far too many individuals and relationships suffer as a result of a lack of understanding of menopause. The UK achieved this in July 2019; Ireland should follow suit.

Early menopause support: Enhanced support for premature ovarian insufficiency (POI), early menopause and cancer-induced early menopause.

We are delighted to see the Department of Health naming the menopause as one of its key areas to focus on in terms of its short-term objectives in improving women's health in Ireland. We are also seeing a much greater number of GPs increasing their knowledge of menopause and ensuring that women get the support that they need. Things are certainly moving in the right direction, but it will take time for women to be fully empowered. This needs to happen through the education system so that ideally the menopause, and perimenopause in particular, will eventually become something that younger women are prepared for well in advance of any symptoms appearing.

A great step forward for Ireland has been the Women's Health Taskforce. Launched by the Department of Health and the National Women's Council of Ireland in 2019, menopause is high on its agenda. It is great to see women being brought together to share and provide their feedback on what needs to change for the better. I am excited to be participating as a menopause advocate, and I hope this initiative will lead to lasting change for the women of Ireland in the future.

In my dream for that future – which is idealistic but not unachievable – it's 2030. Laura sits in her PSHE class listening attentively to the details of menopause and slowly begins to realise that this is why her mum seems more tired and not herself. Anna, Laura's mum, waits in her GP's surgery reading the pamphlet explaining perimenopause in detail and a light bulb goes on. She remembers the national campaign launched a few years back highlighting menopause support in Ireland. It's going to be OK – she understands now what is happening. She has choices. She picks up another booklet, 'Menopause for Your Partner and Family', and decides to bring it home. She chats to her GP, who is a great resource of knowledge on menopause and puts her on the right path. Armed with facts, she leaves the surgery feeling lighter and freer. On returning to work, she books an appointment with the occupational health representative to chat through the existing workplace menopause policy. Within a week she has moved to a desk away from the heat of the window and feels supported by her family and employer.

Essentially, what I would love to see happen is for Irish society to throw out how we've approached menopause so far and start again in a more ambitious way. Menopause should be seen as an essential part of life, an inevitable life stage for women, like any other, from the very beginning. You should start as a teenager, learning at home and at school about menopause. Part of this learning would be a growing acceptance of ageing – this is a crucial hurdle with menopause. We need to change the negative slant on ageing that currently exists to embrace the wisdom we all gain as we get older and positives such as being more comfortable in our own skin.

Then, once a woman enters her childbearing years, and whether or not she has children, there would be education and support from the healthcare system, primary support care teams, doctors and so on, who would all have had in-depth training in menopause in their college years. A routine perimenopause check should become standard – where women receive a full health check covering a breast check, cervical smear, bloodwork, bone density scan (where appropriate), a physiotherapy check to identify bladder health and a gynaecological review, an essential part of which should be vaginal atrophy. Partner support would already be enhanced through secondary-school teaching but should be accessible to all online, via leaflets and through broad national acceptance. This in turn would move the wheels of workplace policies, where menopause would become an implicit part of human resources and/or occupational health.

In the course of my work, I have seen many women whose symptoms have a devastating impact on their lives until they can get a handle on them. There are also many women who, once they develop a personal strategy for addressing their symptoms, really fly. Their creativity takes on a whole new level – they find or revisit a passion and go for it, creating great moments in their lives. It can be a time of great freedom. Daily, I see women who metamorphose into a stronger manifestation of themselves; the analogy of the butterfly is well worn but very appropriate. So many women have gone on new adventures, travelled when they never had before, taken up a new hobby, changed careers, started businesses, returned to college ... the list is endless. The possibilities are endless. The pivotal change is knowing that this is *your* menopause and creating your own toolkit of supports that will help you to thrive through this chapter of life, so that you define your own menopause as opposed to it defining you.

Aisling Grimley is a Dublin-based mother of four daughters. When she hit a hormone speed bump in her late forties, she was shocked to realise how little the topic of menopause was discussed or known. She set up the My Second Spring website in 2013 to open the conversation about menopause and what it means for women, to provide information for the tough times and inspiration for the good ones. My Second Spring aims to help women to make informed decisions about their health at midlife and provide them with a wide variety of approaches to managing symptoms. In 2018, My Second Spring had 2 million visitors worldwide, and is a daily source of support to women in the throes of hormonal havoc. Aisling is an in-demand speaker in corporate workplaces, at events and in media. She is also a founder of The M Word event and The Silk Pillowcase Company.

Catherine O'Keeffe (aka Wellness Warrior.ie) is Ireland's first menopause coach, mother of three boys and a seasoned runner. Following a degree in management, Catherine retrained in complementary medicine and is a self-confessed health geek, a regular contributor to menopause websites and a speaker at health events throughout Ireland and the UK. A former financial services director, Catherine regularly works with corporate clients on menopause support in the workplace. She holds Perimenopause Unplugged events all over Ireland and has established the #MakeMenopauseMatterIreland campaign (an extension of Diane Danzebrink's UK campaign). As a menopause activist, she is a stakeholder in the Women's Health Taskforce, launched by the Department of Health and the National Women's Council of Ireland in 2019. Member of the British Menopause Society, Catherine is also a founder of The M Word event and Brain Health Week, an online virtual summit held annually. Regularly featured in the media, she is author of *The Best Friend's Guide to Anxiety: A Practical Toolkit for Moving Beyond Anxiety at Menopause.*

14

Menopause Is Global

The **Medical Women's International Association** offers an insight into menopause across the world, including contributions from doctors and practitioners in Canada and North America, Italy and Nigeria.

Introduction: Dr Vivien Brown

Dr Vivien Brown is Assistant Professor in the Department of Family and Community Medicine at the University of Toronto. She is the Medical Women's International Association Vice President for North America and leads its initiatives on menopause.

Wherever we are from, we all need to understand the changes in our bodies, the physiology and the transitions as we go from childbearing abilities to menopause. We learn from our mothers and our friends, but we also learn from each other. With the Medical Women's International Association (MWIA), we educate around the world, and our goal is to decrease the stigma, improve daily lives and encourage healthy ageing for our population.

Menopause is not a disease, does not need treatment and does not get 'cured'. We can choose various medications if needed, but this is a choice. Menopause is a process, a time of transition, with lots of changes in a woman's body – not unlike the changes we understand as normal in puberty. I think menopause is an incredible marker in time. It's a time for a woman to review her general health, her lifestyle habits, her symptoms and her abilities. Depending on age and circumstance, there may no longer be the same family demands; often, thankfully, there can be a renewed focus on her own health and making sure she is no longer the very last on her list.

The MWIA was founded in 1919 by Dr Esther Pohl Lovejoy. She was a remarkable doctor, born in 1869, and lived a very active and fulfilling life until her death in her late nineties, in 1967. She was an American physician and public health pioneer, a suffrage activist, a congressional candidate and a central figure in early efforts to organise international medical relief work and public health responsibilities. And it is our organisation today, comprising female medical societies from around the world, present in many countries, on six continents, that continues her work and efforts.

One of the central aims of the MWIA is to offer medical women the opportunity to meet so as to confer upon questions concerning the health and well-being of humanity. It also works to promote the general interest of women in medicine by developing co-operation, friendship and understanding without regard to race, religion or political views, and to address gender-related inequalities in the medical profession. As a global organisation, it also aims to overcome gender-related differences in health and healthcare between women and men, girls and boys throughout the world, and to promote health for all, with a particular interest in women, health and development.

The MWIA has status in various international organisations, including the World Health Organization (WHO), United Nations departments and the UN Economic and Social Council (ECOSOC), and has observer status with the World Medical Association. The initiatives it is involved with around the world range from addressing violence to developing the Safe Childbirth Checklist with WHO and providing birthing kits, and from leadership to work–life balance and sexual harassment. It works on refugee health and ending cervical cancer, and collaborates with the International Menopause Society, as it helps to educate and advocate for women's health in menopause.

With the aims of the organisation and its understanding of the need to both educate and collaborate, MWIA is happy to be part of this book, sharing some knowledge and areas of interest from North America, Italy and Nigeria, around issues of menopause and the effect on women's health.

Dr Marla Shapiro gives an overview of menopause and health in Canada and the US, and shares what has been learned through the Study of Women's Health Across the Nation (SWAN). In Italy, Dr Enrica Ciccarelli has studied early menopause, and reminds us that every woman is different and deserves to be evaluated for her own particular issues, her symptoms and her concerns. Not every case of missed periods means early menopause. Dr Bilqis W. Alatishe-Muhammad shares experiences and studies from Nigeria, and reflects on issues of misunderstanding and long-held beliefs around the ending of periods, and our president, Dr Eleanor Nwadinobi, shares a short personal story about gender and menopausal issues in Nigeria.

Dr Marla Shapiro: Canada and the North American Menopause Society

Past President of the North American Menopause Society, **Dr Shapiro** gives an overview from Canada, where she is Professor in the Department of Family and Community Medicine at the University of Toronto.

I have had the honour of being the Past President of the North American Menopause Society (NAMS). I have also spent the last several years interviewing healthcare professionals in the area of menopausal health as part of an exciting project with NAMS. The videos are available on our website (menopause.org) and cover topics from bone density to sexual health, weight gain at midlife to mood changes, and the latest evidence-based information on hormonal and non-hormonal treatments, cardiovascular health and what is known of the mechanism of hot flushes.

In North America, women are menopausal for more than one-third of their lives. Most women enter menopause somewhere between the ages of 40 and 58; however, the average age for the onset of menopause is 51. Many of my patients will tell me they have finished menopause when their symptoms of hot flushes abate, but I remind them that menopause is not a doorway, but the next phase of life.

The most common symptoms that women complain of – often starting in the perimenopause, when they are still having cycles – are what we call vasomotor symptoms: commonly referred to as hot flushes and night sweats. In addition, one of the more chronic symptoms that presents somewhat later in the menopause is the so-called genitourinary syndrome of menopause, which includes genital symptoms such as dryness and irritation, sexual symptoms related to dryness, lack of lubrication and pain, and urinary symptoms such as urgency, painful urination and recurrent urinary tract infections. Many women are unaware that this syndrome is related to the progressive and chronic loss of oestrogen and think that it is a symptom of ageing.

Many women in North America (research puts the figure at 80 per cent) will experience vasomotor symptoms. A large study called SWAN – the Study of Women's Health Across the Nation – looks at the severity and frequency of these symptoms. Different patterns of onset and persistence have been described in the SWAN data, but we know that the duration of these symptoms for many women is slightly less than eight years, although some women will have symptoms that last more than ten years. Data tells us that a third have severe symptoms more than ten years after menopause and as many as 42 per cent have symptoms after the age of 60. Because of the headline news in 2002 of the findings by the Women's Health Initiative (WHI) study, which looked at the health effects of taking HRT among women in the US, many women became fearful of being treated with hormone therapy and data tells us that as many as 70 per cent of women remain untreated.

We do not completely understand the mechanism of what causes a hot flush, but research is teaching us more every day. It is believed that small changes in core body temperature lead to the sweating, followed often by shivering. These symptoms can be very distressing for women and impact on quality of life. They can also affect sleep quality and duration, leading to impaired daytime functioning. Vasomotor symptoms can also lead to an increase in depressed mood and anxiety. The SWAN study showed us that these symptoms seem to fall into different patterns based on the time from final period and persistence. It also showed that some of these patterns were associated with an increase in cardiovascular disease, but the current information we have does not support treating these symptoms to reduce that risk.

We have also learned about an important concept called the 'timing hypothesis', which tells us what the safest window of treatment opportunity is for women, and the time when it will be effective for symptoms. We know that to be within the first ten years of the onset of menopause; preferably as close to the last menstrual period as possible, and at less than 60 years of age.

The most important message I have for women is to partner with your healthcare provider as an important source of information and education as to how best to manage symptoms. Treatment today is based on the severity of these symptoms, but as NAMS points out in its most recent position statement, treatment must be individualised and based on the particular individual risk factors as well as the personal preferences of that woman. We have a plethora of approved formulations and we encourage ongoing assessment and screening in women. The phrase we are using when it comes to using menopausal hormone therapy for symptomatic women is using the appropriate dose, route and formulation for the appropriate patient for the appropriate length of time.

Women need not suffer because of misinformation and fear.

Dr Enrica Ciccarelli: Studying hormones and younger women in Italy

Based at the Ospedale Martini in Turin, Italy, **Dr Ciccarelli** is a specialist in endocrinology and a member of the Associazione Italiana Donne Medico (AIDM).

Women in Italy experience menopause at an average age of 48.8 years, but 6.3 per cent have early menopause before the age of 40, either spontaneously (1 per cent), or due to medical therapy for tumours or ovary diseases (5.3 per cent), such as chemotherapy and radiotherapy, or treatment for endometriosis. A spontaneous early menopause may be a matter of genetics or related to autoimmune diseases; however, early loss of periods may also be due to a pituitary tumour. These tumours have doubled their incidence during the past thirty years. So, when a younger women stops menstruating, these other possibilities always have to be considered by her doctor or specialist.

Diagnosis can be complex and generally involves looking at the woman's own medical history, family history, symptoms and hormone level tests. To give some insights, I will briefly describe two cases that show two different pathways in diagnosis and therapy, in spite of similar symptoms that the women came to me with.

The first patient I will talk about was aged 36 when she came to see me. She began having periods at 11 and these were regular. There was no family history of early menopause or autoimmune diseases. At 27 years old she developed a thyroid abnormality known as Basedow's disease or Graves' disease and was treated for this; two years later, she was considered cured. At age 34 she was married and wanted to get pregnant, but shortly after this noticed a reduction in her periods. After a year, they disappeared, but without menopausal symptoms. In this kind of case, it is usual to check a woman's hormone levels. My patient's hormonal investigations showed levels that led to a diagnosis of early menopause. She underwent hormone replacement therapy (HRT) for relief of symptoms, but the main issue she was struggling with was infertility, which the hormone therapy could not address. Some years later, she and her husband adopted two children.

My second patient was 34. She started menstruating at age 12 and had always had relatively infrequent periods, with a menstrual cycle of thirty to thirty-five days. There was a family history of hypothyroidism, also known as underactive thyroid (mother), and early menopause (grandmother). At the age of 26, her periods stopped, and she was referred to a gynaecologist who suggested the birth control pill, which can also regulate the menstrual cycle. At the age of 31 she got married and stopped taking the pill, due to headaches. She reported a mild reduction in visual clarity, fatigue and increasing weight. With no periods, the diagnosis of early menopause was suggested by her GP. Six months after stopping the pill, her hormone levels were tested, including for sex hormones, thyroid hormones, adrenal hormones and the stimulating hormones from the brain. The results brought a diagnosis of hypogonadotropic hypogonadism (HH), where the ovaries produce little or no sex hormones because of problems with the hormone-secreting glands in the brain. She also showed other hormone deficiencies linked to this. The MRI brain scan evaluation confirmed the presence of a mass of 4cm in the brain involving critical areas of hormone stimulation.

The patient underwent neurosurgery and this confirmed a meningioma, or tumour on the membranes that surround the brain. Unfortunately, after surgery a large residual tumour was shown. These tumours are usually benign and often the first symptoms patients come with are related to loss of regular pituitary function, or loss of vision. My patient was treated with medications to address the lack of some hormones, but did not want HRT. Pregnancy was advised against because the tumour tissue that was removed showed strong positivity to estradiol and progesterone. In other words, the tumour that remained could grow due to the stimulation of hormones, so pregnancy could endanger the patient.

Menstruation ceasing in younger women may raise possible different diagnoses – it could be due to early menopause or it could be HH. As the cases above show, the symptoms the women presented with may not be significant in reaching the correct diagnosis; family history is also not necessarily of help. Menopausal symptoms are not always present, and can be misleading. It is the hormonal diagnosis that is essential for the right therapy. In particular, checking the levels of gonadotropins, estradiol and prolactin is essential, as the balance of hormones in the body is altered at different times in our lives. A correct diagnosis is essential for the appropriate therapy, which is usually HRT for early menopause and surgery for removing a pituitary tumour.

Both of these patients had wanted to become pregnant and the discovery of infertility was their major source of distress. Depression also had a large impact on their lives, their marriages and their future goals. All women need appropriate care and as doctors we strive to focus on each patient, their age, their issues and their specific circumstances, as not all cases of lack of periods are truly a diagnosis of menopause.

Dr Bilqis W. Alatishe-Muhammad: Perspectives from Nigeria

Dr Bilqis W. Alatishe-Muhammad is a Public Health Physician (Senior Registrar) at the University of Ilorin teaching hospital, with a particular interest in social and rehabilitative health.

I have a special interest in the subject of menopause. So much so that I wrote and published a booklet in August 2018 entitled *Menopause: The*

'Super Adult' Woman's Life. Sharing my experiences as a contribution to a book meant to serve the global network of womenfolk is an opportunity that I appreciate. Every woman needs to understand that 'menopause is an inevitable part of the ageing process for every woman who is opportune to live through that period of life'.

As a clinician, I have interacted with several patients who often walk into the clinic *only* to ask questions about menopause. It should be emphasised that cessation of menstrual flow is not the only event in menopause. Hence menopause, as simple as it may seem, needs to be differentiated from other health conditions that share similar features. In medical school, a classmate stopped menstruating at the age of 25. That would be a big surprise to anyone. She had just got married, she wasn't pregnant, but she did not menstruate for up to eighteen months. Investigations later revealed that she had premature ovarian failure (which is a medical cause of premature menopause).

I have also seen patients who have non-specific complaints about a generalised discomfort, without really conceptualising its relationship to the onset of a change in menstrual pattern. This occurs commonly in the perimenopausal period and only gets unravelled by an experienced medical practitioner who does not leave anything to chance. I am used to comments like: 'Doctor! I cannot explain how I am feeling. There is this hotness flowing down through my body, as if there is fire moving round it. My head is aching, my joints are aching. In fact, Doctor, I do not understand my body any more.'

Studies have shown that the menopausal age in Nigeria is comparable to that of other populations and the manifestation of menopausal symptoms in Nigerian women may constitute a significant health burden. Healthcare providers should therefore be knowledgeable about the manner in which Nigerian women perceive menopausal symptoms.

Some of the research done in Nigeria looking at issues around menopause has been conducted among the Yoruba tribe. It revealed an average menopausal age of 48 years, with no relationship established between menopausal age and various biosocial factors such as age of menarche, social class, number of pregnancies, smoking and place of residence. Many of the women surveyed presented with symptoms such as joint pains and hot flushes, with only 42 per cent of them still practising sexual intercourse.

Nigerian women see old age as a stage in a woman's life when she is accorded respect and is regarded as an embodiment of wisdom. Older women are seen as custodians of the culture of the community they live in and it is believed that women become wiser when menstruation ends and thereafter can rise in social status and even assume leadership positions. On the other hand, many communities believe that menopause is a disease and the woman can infect her husband with such disease. They have the assumption that it is a spell from witchcraft. They also believe it leads to loss of weight and it must begin only at the age of 50.

Another study showed that only a few of the respondents had a reasonable idea about why women menstruate. Most saw menstruation only as a means of cleansing the dirtiness in them – so it is important that a woman observes her menstruation every month. In such cultural settings, where menstrual bleeding is highly valued as a sign of health and youth, menopausal women may welcome even abnormal bleeding as a sign of continued fertility and thus fail to seek necessary medical care.

Only a very few women were said to have viewed menopause as a fact of life which had to come at its right time, and as an opportunity for them to meet their religious obligations more regularly and fully.

In this part of the world, belonging to social groups is one of the ways in which women adjust to the menopausal stage. Many others engage themselves in business, or revive an activity in which they showed talent or had some training in their youth. This was also reflected in a study where most of the women were seen to belong to one or more social groups, so offering support to individual members.

A key objective of a public enlightenment on menopause is to dispel as many misconceptions and myths as possible. Menopause is one of those health conditions associated with many such misconceptions in Nigeria. Many younger perimenopausal women, who still want to have more children, usually present with negative attitudes towards menopause, like depression. At menopause, sexual intercourse is often seen as an abominable act. Studies in Nigeria have well established the prevalence of the notion that postmenopausal sex causes ill health. Such deep-seated cultural beliefs may unfortunately encourage infidelity on the part of husbands who have sexual desires but are unwilling to be the cause of their wives' medical problems. In addition to this, most of the women surveyed expressed their lack of interest in sex and reported that their sexual frequency had diminished. This loss of interest in sex seems to be directly proportional to the women's age. Many women also claim not to know about HRT and those who knew were sceptical about its safety.

Some women also claim that they don't have a forum where they can be counselled about menopause. As well as providing health guidance, having a Well Woman Clinic for women around this age could help in dispelling traditional myths and taboos that are prevalent around this period of human development in the female gender. It could also correct the practice of sexual abstinence at menopause and the misconception of menopause as a disease.

Dr Eleanor Nwadinobi: A personal encounter

President of the MWIA, **Dr Eleanor Nwadinobi is** an accomplished doctor and a gender and human rights consultant who has won many accolades.

In the south-east of Nigeria, the kolanut is presented as a symbol of welcome, but only to men. A small ceremony is conducted whereby the guest blesses the kolanut with prayers, breaks it by snapping it and then shares it with men and women in the gathering to eat.

On one occasion, I accompanied my aunt, who was in her late sixties, on an advocacy visit to a man in authority. He welcomed us by presenting the customary kolanut to my aunt. He announced that he was doing this as a mark of respect because he considered her to be a 'man' since she was postmenopausal. My aunt took this as a great insult, whereas the host expected her to feel honoured at being given the respect which is the exclusive preserve of men. In his words: 'You have reached a stage in your life [menopause] where I consider you to be a man.'

15

An Act of Renaming and Reclaiming

Journalist and broadcaster **Caryn Franklin** looks at how we can address society's unrealistic obsession with youth and negative projections of the maturing feminine appearance by reframing the postmenopause picture.

It's a few years since I first wrote about my raw experience of menopause in an article for *Refinery29*. At that time, I spoke about how I battled with a near-constant brain fug that led me to wonder whether I was suffering from early onset dementia, and being cast adrift by a tidal wave of anxiety. What I did not know at that point was that the menopause would be the gift that would keep on giving. In forcing me to stop and listen to my body and myself in a way that I had not done before, I began to reclaim and reframe my life. But that was all to come. Telling my story in 2018, I wrote:

> Life had suddenly become very confusing ... one minute I was cruising a marvellously lit highway in a 4x4. The next, without noticing I had taken a wrong turn, I was bouncing down a dark dirt track in a broken-down banger.
>
> 'How did I get here?' I kept asking, 'and' (more to the point) 'how can I get out?' I was used to problem-solving and multitasking. Having

worked in the fashion industry for more than 30 years, while raising a family, running a business and campaigning for a variety of women's issues, I had not signed up for this chaos. I quickly became anxious about what each new day would hold ...

Industry knowledge evaporated and I found myself unable to remember names, events and dates. My vocabulary shrank too. At home both daughters would play guessing games to get me to the end of my sentence, and my youngest still reminds me of the day I forgot her name ...

Meanwhile, I was medicating myself with generous amounts of Cabernet Sauvignon each evening. Anaesthetising anxiety this way helped me limp on for a bit longer, clinging to the remnants of my previously ordered existence. Then I made an important decision. I stopped and stood still. 'What do I need to understand?' I asked myself, having read enough to realise that female bodies are powerful intuitive barometers and mine was trying to tell me something. This is what I learned.

The voice was right. I was finished. But an ending of the way I had been living would be a good thing. Since leaving education I had put in very long hours building a career. As a dedicated parent and partner, I routinely put others first, which meant racing through my life overachieving for others and under-prioritising me. Exhausted and running on empty, letting go of my expectations of me would be the first positive move.

I started to decline an occasional paid job that didn't suit, pursuing serenity over superfluous funds, and embraced a new chapter in my academic education, which required time and space. I embarked on a new way of framing my skills and talents, thinking about the bigger picture as I celebrated my strengths and focused on the positives, while gracefully accepting my limitations ... finally. Trusting this joyous momentum, a giving of birth to myself afresh, I began to clear out old thinking: from now on, instinct would be my guide.

'She's let herself go.' I've written about this over the years – the way in which such statements perpetuate an unrealistic obsession with clinging on to youth and a negative framing of the maturing feminine appearance. All of which continues to see shelves stuffed full of anti-ageing balms and hair dye. Well, I'm still not buying it.

Is beauty advertising a guilty pleasure or an oppressive voice of denunciation? The formula, practically unchanged over time, reproduces a thin, young, white, able-bodied woman, sleek of mane with straight nose, wet, pouty lips and marvellous dentistry, looking ever so slightly pre-orgasmic. That she will be standing next to a wind machine to be recorded, as photographers like to say, 'in the moment between moments', and this shot will have taken most of the day to capture, is not at the forefront of our minds when we consider the product and its claims. Nor is the fact that within the digital file containing her image, the model we see will be airbrushed to within an inch of her papillary dermis, despite being too young to display even one of the seven signs of ageing we're routinely told to guard against.

And before our model makes it to a giant billboard her likeness, now devoid of authentic selfhood, will have endured further levels of scrutiny and mechanical manipulation. Beauty porn is proudly out in the open. Its presence has conditioned and socialised all who view femininity through this limiting lens to unknowingly objectify and diminish those who do not conform. As women we know it makes for degrading viewing, but it's highly compelling just the same. And we all want to believe in transformation, don't we?

'But surely if you're paying top dollar for a cream, you're getting something special?' 'Yes,' I say, not wanting to devalue the random request for insight. 'It can be expensive to make a special shoot with a top photographer, a special supermodel or celebrity and an entourage of special executives in an exotic location and then plaster the special results to the billboards of the Western world. And how do you think they pay for that?'

But is there something bigger than the storytelling itself? Psychology confirms what female scholars know: repetition of unachievable beauty images creates appearance anxiety. It also dispenses powerful propaganda for a belief system that does not honour authentic female process: namely the passing of youthful daughter, into nurturing mother and wise authoritative grandmother. There is little in our culture to iconise female maturity, but there is plenty to denigrate it.

My daughters have a feminist mother who has decoded mass-media babble since Barbie infiltrated our house in sneaky birthday present mode decades ago. They celebrate the insights they have accrued and deliberately sought their own knowledge. As children, I and my sisters were not so well prepared, but then there was less beauty assault on little girl brains for our mother to protect against. The Kate Hepburns, and later the Brigitte Bardots, embodied a certain wholesome reality, or at least a photographic honesty. With nothing more than a pot of Nivea and a Box Brownie to record them in a sepia soft finish, these beautiful women aged in their own way. If Bardot would later choose to live life in the great outdoors, prioritising animals, not sun block, then so be it. As a result, our mother, a beautiful woman, never obsessed about 'getting older' – it was something that everybody did together.

Fifty years on, we're wrapped up in a post-feminist, 'women buying it for themselves' euphoria. Now anti-ageing treatments range from obscure ingredients in fancy pots and lunchtime 'tweakment' procedures to the full-blown cutting, pumping, stuffing and sewing of tissues – the results of which adorn marketing imagery on personal screens inside the home. There are also invitations in our magazines from beauty factories to undergo the cut. With this encouragement reaching saturation point in our brains, are those of us with the funds prompted, triggered and traumatised into appearance compliance? Women may have turned the gaze on themselves, to become their own harshest critics, but this is only part of a condition that acculturates mass-media audiences to consume female beauty as a thing of itself.

The consumption of women as aesthetic service providers in public spaces has normalised a sense of entitlement by the viewer to see narrow beauty standards upheld. It is not just about the tabloid shaming of celebrity ageing and the disappearance of our elder stateswomen on TV; female image is a workplace issue too. In demanding uncomfortable dress codes for women only, companies confirm that who we are, what we know and what we stand for carries less significance than how we present. Do we pass the grade? Are we acceptable? A 2013 UK Girlguiding study found that 87 per cent of girls and young women surveyed between the ages of 11 and 21 believed that women were judged more on their appearance than their ability. In 2017, writing in UK *Grazia*, journalist Barbara Bourland recounted the story of a friend who prioritised Botox above her rent because she was afraid of getting fired for being ugly. Women of colour negotiate additional appearance racism in career environments, steeling themselves against unwanted touching of, and commentary about, their hair on a daily basis. The intolerance of dreadlocks has even been legally defended by a US Circuit Court of Appeals to uphold white supremacist employer recruitment prejudice.

It's easy to see how, when appearance becomes an evaluative gaze by those in power, we are bullied into thinking we aren't enough. Business culture is there to confirm this by paying us less. The National Women's Law Center has calculated that in 2017 white, non-Hispanic women earned 77 cents for every dollar a man did, while Black women earned only 61 cents for every dollar, based on figures from US Census Bureau comparing median earnings of those in year-round, full-time employment.

Throughout our lives we have become familiar with a kind of gender appraisal, represented by the popular cartoon of a workplace board meeting. In this illustration, the only woman round the table of men is told by her boss: 'Nice idea but let's wait until a man suggests it.' I'm smiling as I write. It's ridiculous but true, and throughout my long career in womenswear, there have been many tables and many white male voices during my repeated challenge to the fashion industry's dependence on the thin, white, young model as a one-size-fits-all marketing ideal. In fact, I have agitated, advocated, remonstrated and rallied in favour of a broader range of body and beauty ideals in size, race and age representation for decades; this last one being particularly important to business given that women over 40 have four times as much to spend on one garment. And I have presented a variety of female customer-centric needs to do with fit, product and protocol. Benefiting from both race and class privilege, I can only imagine how much bigger the wall of indifference might have been without this unearned social ranking. I am humbled by the amount of energy marginalised women must allocate in pursuit of making themselves heard in these environments and review my own historical complacency that race, class and health privilege afforded me. Small and large shifts have at last begun to happen in my industry. One particular triumph pertaining to realistic representation of women, and preceded by regular dissent from me as an employee on a longstanding fashion events platform, came only after the ascension of a woman to the position of managing director to the firm. Proof that our vital presence in leadership is needed for significant progress.

But even now in a dark tunnel unlit by stories and comradery of menopausal women before me in workplace battle cry, the void continues. Passing as species neutral, devoid of hormonal payload or laments about the grossly inequitable parenting and domestic obligations borne by our sex, has become standard practice for many of us. This along with the physical work our bodies perform: menstruation, conception, abortion, miscarriage, pregnancy, birth and menopause is shouldered by women at work in private. What our biology compels us to accomplish has been hushed up by us all, lest it affect perception of our gender's output as single-minded or focused and dedicated workers. The lack of learning and pointers for new process, therefore, as I reach the crest of my own sexual labour, is stark.

Some of us have made our mark, forced our presence, and risen through the ranks with the glare of an unforgiving gender spotlight on our proficiency. And we have made it our business to reach out to other women and pull them up. So why then did our mentors agree to walk this stretch of shadowy passage alone and in silence? It will be a question, disquieting in its complexity, that mutes my own workplace voice too. Then I understand. It would not do, as we reach leadership status or governing position with the opportunity to deliver a more emotionally sustainable workplace for the women who follow, to expose our biochemical shake-up. The potential for sabotaging all that has been achieved seems too great to risk.

So, I realise why women before me chose to remain quiet about their perimenopausal turmoil. I have only written about my experience after safely reaching the other side. During it, I did not declare temporary loss of mental capacity either. Survival instinct would be one way to explain this reflex. Social science explains it other ways. Studies looking at male-dominated environments and cultures found that women were more likely to anticipate gender-based rejection. This was attributed to 'rejection sensitivity', as a result of being historically excluded along with other devalued or minority groups. In 2012, researchers also found that, in anticipation of negative outcomes linked to gender-based rejection, women chose to mute or self-silence.

In another experiment, researchers manipulated body focus by having women and men try on a swimsuit before returning to their original street clothes as part of what they believed to be a shopping survey. At a later point, a maths test was undertaken and measured against previous grades. In 1998 researchers found that for women only, the experience of focusing on the body consumed important attentional resources and resulted in diminished mathematical performance. In other words, women are triggered into body-image preoccupation when they are reminded to focus on their bodies, and, let's be frank, this is almost always, given popular culture obsession with female appearance.

It is not now, nor has it ever been the case that women deliver lesser workplace competency than men. Only that, within the structures we exist in, our lived experience of self is frequently destabilised. Beauty ideologies accompany women throughout their lives, but it is as we age that we become doubly exposed to pressure and expectations.

Let's spell it out. Like some grim brainwashing torment, the trauma of being set up to evaluate our physical selves against unethical unachievable white ideals, constantly reminded of our imperfect or racially incompatible appearance when we are young, and gaslit as we begin to age about what we will lose, not only interferes with the ability of women to think straight, it destroys our sense of entitlement to just be. Our gender has been groomed to self-objectify while beauty corporations grow rich. And have we, in the process of consuming femininity as a set of unrealistic appearance goals, become blind to our internal exquisiteness?

I recognise any cis or trans woman's right to do what she wishes with her body and her appearance. Now with long grey hair, it's my choice to present as accomplished and sagacious. I don't play the patriarchal game of defining myself as decorative dressing in a man-made world. Maybe this has helped me to embrace the privilege of age with its intellectual and experiential gifts. I do believe that if we can stop focusing solely on exteriors and start embracing personhood, postmenopause becomes a position of status and composure.

And I am not alone in knowing that women have much to contribute. Research by Korn Ferry Institute looked at data from 55,000 participants in ninety countries from 2011 to 2015, correlating emotional intelligence with effective leadership and management, and found that women were higher scorers than men in eleven out of twelve emotional and social intelligence categories and therefore 86 per cent more likely to behave with emotional intelligence beneficial to workplace productivity. Yet we suppress our voices in the unfounded belief that we are lesser, such is the conditioning women receive throughout their lives. Stepping up now, to influence, to push back, is paramount. The planet needs us. The next generation needs us: 'Exploitative male systems may have pushed us all so very close to disaster without precedent in our history,' notes Barbara G. Walker in her 1985 book *The Crone*.

As my workplace identity continues to unfold, and choosing strategic contraction where I can in order to amplify my energy and voice, I celebrate and promote stories of female agency and empowerment. These are the truths that have spurred me on, but I am thankful for the privilege to action my own passage; a tour guide and sightseer in one. So, what more do I wish to know on this voyage of discovery?

In pre-historical narratives, we find gnarly elder stateswomen who exist beyond the confines of commerce and politics to embody a multidimensional, all-seeing wisdom. Woman as Goddess, Tribal Elder, Oracle and Shaman presents as mystical being, harnessing and recharging her power through effortless connectivity with the earth, the wind and the skies to celebrate the cycle of life and the miracle of nature. From Nana Buluku, the West African mother goddess attributed with the creation of the world, Baba Yaga, the Russian mistress of magic, Kali, the Indian goddess of destruction and rebirth, to Ereshkigal, the Sumerian goddess of the underworld, to name but a few, I want sight of these missing crones in our modern world. I want our daughters to watch us age and know that entering the society of cronehood positions us for the highest office; a venerated state of wisdom and output.

My *Collins Concise Dictionary Plus* consists of over 1,500 pages. While some entries run into paragraphs, one line is given for the crone. From this hefty tome we learn only that she is a 'witch-like old woman'. Spinster fares no better: 'An unmarried woman; a woman beyond the age of marriage'; and to finish, 'a woman who spins thread for a living'. At least feminist history can be relied upon to lay out the fuller picture of female selfhood across many cultures. From Amazons and Assyrian war queens, to scientists and, yes, spinsters – who, by the way, engaged in agriculture, animal husbandry, spinning and weaving to take charge of their own livelihoods as respected traders of product – we can know women were so much more than assessment of their relationship to men. As Rosalind Miles points out in her 1988 *The Women's History of The World*, 'all is lost, when history concentrates on men only'.

Which it does. With Christianity centralising masculine agendas and ideologies, and scapegoating all the daughters of Eve as sinners in need of control, innocent beautiful virgins might be tolerated as wife material. But angry middle-aged women, making unwanted interventions in an oppressive culture that continues to undermine female wisdom, would be denounced as ugly witches or heretics and brutally dispatched. Hundreds of years later, the quest for gender parity and fairness remains, and growing old without self-reproach is one deliciously subversive act all women can embrace.

So, do we 'let ourselves go'? Or are we simply releasing ourselves from unreasonable structures and hierarchies as a vital part of the process? This shifting and discarding of a previous self may well be accompanied by turbulence or unrest, but compensation awaits. You will find it, once out the other side, in the form of a new selfhood and a new voice. Surrendering to something bigger than you does not need to be an act of powerlessness, it can be an education and an enlightenment. We can prepare ourselves as best we can by seeking out others who have been or are on the same journey, as listening to other women's stories when I was at my lowest helped me to see the way. We can also equip ourselves by seeking more tranquillity, more sleep, a healthy diet, supportive friends, and treating ourselves with the kindness we are due. Let's afford the rearrangement of our biochemistry with the respect it deserves. In doing so, we can rename and reclaim post-menopause as an ushering in of discovery, creativity and prestige. Thus, our hormonal uproar becomes that much-needed and powerful challenge to a world that needs our thunder.

Caryn Franklin MBE is a former fashion editor and co-editor of *i-D magazine*; a BBC primetime TV fashion presenter and broadcaster, now commentator and activist. Her projects have involved international design names and everyday users of fashion as well as refugees in battle zones, garment workers in free-trade-zone slums, mental health and body-image experts, MPs and government. She has written for numerous magazines, newspapers and websites, produced four books and authored many TV shows and documentaries on fashion, as well as co-created groundbreaking campaigns such as Fashion Targets Breast Cancer and multi-award-winning All Walks Beyond the Catwalk. In recent years, and with an MSc in Applied Psychology investigating selfhood, objectification, inclusivity and bias, Caryn has consulted with corporate leadership initiatives and progressive educational institutions. She is a Visiting Professor of Diverse Selfhood at Kingston School of Art. Contact her on Instagram @franklinonfashion.

16

Our Unspoken Needs: The Women of Afghanistan

Award-winning filmmaker, presenter and activist **Arzu Qaderi** has filmed and interviewed women throughout Afghanistan about their lives, and uses this to give voice to what is for many the unspoken topic of menopause and women's health.

Menopause is a highly sensitive topic in Afghanistan, as in the Western hemisphere and beyond. Many women feel silenced and degraded by cultures that see the changing female body as useless. In Muslim countries, the menopause, like menstruation, carries particular negative connotations; the menopause is not a topic that is spoken about openly and neither is it discussed in private, woman-to-woman conversations.

The position of women in Afghanistan has undergone dramatic changes in the past three decades. Following years of occupation by the Soviet Union and intervention by other countries, from 1992 Afghanistan was engulfed by a devastating civil war, with the Taliban eventually taking control in 1996. This was the beginning of five years of severely reduced rights for women. Education for girls was banned, as were many types of work for women. The burqa was obligatory, and women could be punished for transgressions such as forgetting to wear it outside the home.

There have been significant improvements since the signing of the Bonn Agreement in 2001 that set up the Afghan interim government. Millions of girls and women have been educated, and some are taking leading roles. More than a quarter (28 per cent) of Afghanistan's MPs are female, according to 2019 figures from the Inter-Parliamentary Union, the global organisation of national parliaments. The reported experience of Afghan women shows that they are also setting up businesses, pioneering new areas of activity for women and are involved in the arts, sport, community initiatives and medicine.

However, problems such as low female literacy, high maternal mortality and violence against women are still of great concern. Less than 30 per cent of women over the age of 15 can read and write, according to 2018 figures from UNESCO, compared with 55 per cent of men. The maternal mortality rate is estimated as 638 per 100,000 live births (the comparable numbers in the UK and US are 7 and 19 respectively), based on 2017 figures that the World Bank Group has brought together from WHO, UNICEF and UNFPA. Early in 2020, the Afghan Women's Network reported an increased level of violence, insecurity and criminal attacks in the country. It had previously stated that:

> Deprivation of the right to education, harassment at educational places, work places, on the streets; moreover, forced and child marriages, deprivation of rights to inheritance and dowry, sexual violence, rape, murder, kidnapping, slander, cyberbullying, exchange marriages, desert courts, threats and intimidation, forced divorce, no charity, beatings ... are common violence in Afghanistan.

In April 2019, Islamic State attacked the Afghan communications ministry in Kabul, where working women had previously been appreciative of the childcare facilities, while in May that year the Taliban killed nine people at the offices of aid agency Counterpart International. A Taliban representative said the agency was targeted because it was involved in 'harmful Western activities', including the 'inter-mixing' of women and men.

Afghanistan has a relatively young population. Average life expectancy is estimated as 64 years, rising to 66 for women (based on 2017 figures aggregated from sources including the UN and national statistical offices). The country's high rate of infant mortality skews these averages, however, and a significant and growing number of women will live into and beyond menopause. Estimates from the United Nations Population Division suggest that about 68 per cent of Afghan women born in 2017 will reach the age of 65.

Traditionally, Afghanistan has been a patriarchal and patrilineal society, and is still largely so, particularly in conservative rural areas. After menopause, a woman might be referred to as a 'respected old woman', or else as 'mother of ...' (*madar-i ...*) her eldest son, or daughter if she had no sons.

Academic research on attitudes to menopause and menstruation among Afghan women has so far largely been conducted among migrant and refugee women living in Western countries, such as Australia and Canada. Research published in 2019 by Professor Jane Ussher and a team from the Western Sydney University quoted one participant as saying, 'your period, it ejects a lot of toxins from your body ... it may not be a good thing when it dries up'. Although the researchers reported that for many in their study, menstruation was seen as shameful or impure, women may also traditionally be regarded as more vulnerable to ill health when their periods stop, because of their 'purifying' aspect. The study found from the Afghan women interviewed that here – as in many other countries – women's health, and in particular reproductive and sexual health, remains a taboo subject, often surrounded by silence and secrecy. However, from an Islamic legal point of view, as discussed in the *Encyclopedia of Women and Islamic Cultures*, older women have greater freedom of movement and action; they may be able to enter situations that would be forbidden to younger women and be subject to less scrutiny. They are not bound by the same rules of purification and abstinence from prayer as menstruating women, and so potentially can be more active in their worship.

As an Afghan-born woman who grew up in Germany, Arzu Qaderi wanted to explore female empowerment and the ongoing fight for equality across the world. In her work, she places her focus on women who come from marginalised backgrounds. For her first documentary, *My Afghan Diary*, filmed in Kabul, she wanted to hear what life was really like for women in Afghanistan – going beyond the stereotypical media depictions – in order to share their richly nuanced stories far and wide, and to find the role models that other women might look to. The film includes interviews with multitalented women working within the media sector who, despite the odds, have succeeded in Afghanistan, which remains a patriarchal society suffering from ongoing conflict.

During filming, Arzu also spoke to women activists in Afghanistan who tirelessly campaign for what they believe in. Among those she met during the filming are advocate for women's political participation Diba Naikpay and human rights activist Mawloda Tamana Nazari.

In this chapter, Arzu and some of her interviewees and contacts set out key challenges facing Afghan women. Menopause in this country is not yet a subject that has emerged from taboo status. In Afghanistan, the focus is on securing a more stable future without sacrificing women's rights, on political participation, on countering violence against women, and on women's health more widely, in particular access to health facilities and medicines.

Arzu Qaderi: What led me to film *My Afghan Diary*

Arzu Qaderi is an award-winning documentary filmmaker, presenter and activist. She has worked extensively in fashion and launched her presenting career in 2012 when she hosted her own weekly fashion news show, *Fresh Cuts*. Arzu has received a citation from the federal government of Ottawa, Canada, for her contributions to this industry. Born in Afghanistan, she grew up in Germany and filmed her first documentary, *My Afghan Diary*, on her return to Kabul. The film has won multiple awards, including 'Best Documentary' in the Festival del Cinema di Salerno and 'Best Short Documentary' in both the Jaipur International Film Festival and the Mediterranean Film Festival Cannes. It has been screened in Canada, London, Chile and her home city of Hamburg. Arzu has also given speeches about the importance of women's health in Afghanistan and received an honorary award at the Women Appreciating Women Awards.

When Audre Lorde said: 'I am not free while any woman is unfree, even when her shackles are very different from my own,' she spoke to me and billions of other women across the globe of our collective legacy; we all have an immense responsibility to each other.

We have come so far since the first known gathering devoted to women's rights in the US, the Seneca Falls Convention held in July 1848. The two women who organised that gathering were Elizabeth Cady Stanton and

Lucretia Mott, and Stanton put together the famous declaration stating: 'We hold these truths to be self-evident: that all men and women are created equal.' This birthed the suffrage movement, whose fierce campaigning led to the recognition of women's right to vote in America a hundred years ago, in 1920. Now it is up to the next generations – both women and men – to carry on this important work, and I have devoted my life to spreading this message of positivity.

These beliefs are what led me to film *My Afghan Diary*, when I returned to Kabul for the first time since my birth there. I wanted to truly make a positive contribution to the depiction of Afghan women in the media and so I decided to take it into my own hands, filming my documentary in September 2018.

A major difficulty I faced is the ban and ongoing censorship on filming publicly in Afghanistan. Photography is also banned. I was aware that this passion project was a huge risk to my livelihood and those of the people working with me, so I kept to a very small team and all details were extremely confidential – we could not afford to make any errors because the potential risks were high. In the opening sequence of the film there is striking footage of the deserted streets of Kabul, filmed out of a car window, with me hiding and using a handheld camera in the back of the vehicle. Our equipment had to be inconspicuous and our interviews were set up on the day of filming, with locations kept secret. At the time I was aware that I had to get it done, or no one else would bring these valuable stories to the big screen. I was truly amazed at the inner strength that these women conveyed and what they confided in me; they still inspire me.

Making contact with the women was a two-step process. Due to the sensitive nature of the subject matter, I had to approach them through someone they knew and trusted. Setting up the location was also a private and confidential matter – one of the locations, Kabul Theatre, was bombed only a few days after we filmed there – so keeping the project between a small group of people was essential to all of our safety. I spoke to young women and mature women with years of experience behind them, although a recurring theme across all age ranges is the friction with male family members when pursuing ambitious dreams, due to the expectations placed on women to not work and to stay at home. At first, inevitably, there was a reluctance to discuss personal areas, as the possible backlash if family members were to see these interviews could affect family relations. My approach as an interviewer prioritises empathy and, despite the private nature of Afghan women, they understood that I was providing them with a safe platform to share their personal experiences.

Throughout the film I had the opportunity to speak with many strong, pioneering women. Women like Soosan Firooz, one of the first female rappers in Afghanistan, who voices her questions about society through singing and rapping; Laila Hamdard, who proudly proclaims that theatre is her life and shares amazing pictures of the productions she has led; and the passionate Selly Ghafoori, who is also a devoted actress with a bright future ahead of her.

A universal theme for all the women I met and interviewed in Afghanistan was that of continuing to follow their dreams despite the outside world not always being in harmony with them: something that women in the Western world can identify with too. Sediqa Tamkin, for example, is an artist who through her insightful words highlights the balancing act of being a mother, a wife and an artist – and remaining true to all of those identities.

Menopause should be a topic that is openly spoken of, without shame, since we all as women will go through it. As a younger woman, I have not yet fully explored the subject of menopause within my own family or friendship circle, but I am surrounded by supportive family and friends with whom I am always able to speak openly – a privilege for which I am very grateful.

In 2012 I gave a speech for the European Campaign for Human Rights, highlighting the extraordinarily high risk of dying during pregnancy in Afghanistan, which has the highest maternal mortality rate in the world. This war-torn country has been left with a damaged healthcare system that is severely understaffed, an issue that still remains, with a worrying lack of maternal healthcare in large parts of the country. These are all still current issues and it is imperative to continue raising awareness about them, to improve the collective health of Afghan women and to help reduce the preventable maternal and child deaths that occur at a high rate.

This current generation of women are, however, forging their own paths and working together towards a more equal Afghanistan. I am hopeful regarding the representation of women in Afghan politics, where they are boldly putting women's issues at the forefront and working tirelessly towards a brighter future for all.

Diba Naikpay: The importance of politics and women's participation

A youth outreach assistant in the Women and Youth Department of the Free and Fair Election Forum of Afghanistan (FEFA), **Diba** is an English Literature graduate from Kabul University and trained journalist. She is also an active member of the Men Supporting Women's Rights (MSWR)/ Counterpart organisation.

The political participation of Afghan women is a concerning issue. When the Taliban regime collapsed in 2001, Afghanistan, along with the international community, made attempts to establish a democratic state in the country – for all citizens to have equal rights and duties in a democratic system. The participants in the Bonn conference raised the issue of women's participation and fair representation of all ethnic and religious groups in an interim government, and women's participation in the political democratic process is a must.

After the collapse of the Taliban, women have been able to have active roles in the government framework. Currently, women are working as ministers, governor, deputy ministers, chairperson and members of parliament. They are also owners of small businesses and chairs of public and private universities. Based on the Bonn Agreement, the interim government of Afghanistan established the Ministry of Women's Affairs. The first Minister of Women's Affairs was Mrs Sima Samar, who led the ministry from 2001 until 2002.

The Ministry of Women's Affairs is responsible for monitoring and making sure that women's legitimate rights are considered and observed in the government's areas of activity. Over the seventeen years since it was founded, many other organisations have been established to work for women's rights, such as the Afghan Women's Network, Voice of Afghan Women and MSWR/Counterpart.

The vision of FEFA is to work through partnerships, citizen participation, good governance and professional programmes to enhance transparency and accountability in democratic processes. FEFA's Women and Youth Outreach Department works for women's political rights and women's participation in the political process. FEFA established the Women's Political Rights Advocacy Group (WPRAG) to review women's problems. WPRAG is made up of members of parliament, media, electoral commission representatives, women's rights activists and company chief executives. Our aim is to work for women and discover the problems and barriers that they face in political participation; we try to find solutions from our advocacy groups and share with stakeholders.

There are a number of reasons why women's participation in politics is less than it could and needs to be. These range from female illiteracy and lack of belief in women's abilities, to home responsibilities, harmful cultural traditions, women's economic dependence and a patriarchal culture. Families can also be unaware of the political process, especially elections. There is a shortage of female police for maintaining the security of elections and a lack of female staff at the polling centres, which can also be remote. Electoral fraud and corruption, and a lack of support for women, are also issues, plus continued security threats and the political circumstances. The National Unity Government and the law enforcement institutions are recommended to undertake the necessary steps for eliminating these challenges.

However, despite difficult circumstances, women have managed to prove their significant role in Afghan society and politics. Encouraging their even greater participation in all aspects of the political process, in my opinion, the Afghan government has made significant efforts to develop a legal framework enshrining equality between women and men. This has to be implemented at all levels of society by dismantling the remaining practices that prevent the full and equal participation of women.

Noorjahan Akbar: Addressing violence against women

Women's rights advocate and author **Noorjahan Akbar** has worked with Afghan and global organisations focusing on women's empowerment and ending gender-based violence, and has led nationwide campaigns and protests. She runs Free Women Writers, a collective of activists and writers in Afghanistan and the diaspora, and has published in *Al Jazeera* and the *New York Times*. She has featured on *Forbes*'s 'Women Changing the World', Fast Company's 'League of Extraordinary Women', and *The Daily Beast*'s 'Women Who Shake the World' lists.

One in three women around the world has faced physical or sexualised violence – and that doesn't include emotional, financial or verbal violence. These women are not mere numbers, but people we know. In Afghanistan, the numbers are even more staggering. While it's hard to find dependable and current statistics about the rates of violence, especially in rural areas, we know from anecdotes, and I know from working in this field for more than a decade, that there is rarely any woman whose life has not been touched by gendered violence in some way. If we grew up in safe, loving homes, we were likely to face harassment on the streets. If our homes and streets were safe, we faced harassment at the workplace or at our educational institutions. Even if now we are in safety, many of us continue to deal with the trauma of physical and sexualised violence that we faced as children, teens and young adults.

This is why in 2016, Free Women Writers, a collective I created with women writers, activists and artists from Afghanistan, published the book *You Are Not Alone*, first in Persian and Pashto and then in English for Afghan women facing violence at home. *You Are Not Alone* is a short guide to provide women facing violence in Afghanistan with legal tips as well as emotional support. Written after four years of research and speaking with survivors of violence through our platforms and in conversation, this book hopes to help women heal from the violence they have faced or free themselves from violence they are facing.

Through this book we want to let fellow Afghan women know that they are not alone, that they have a sisterhood that is rooting for them and willing to listen to their stories and believe them; that they are not to blame for the violence they face, and that they have the power to overcome violence. We use the book also as an opportunity to dispel some of the myths that surround violence (such as that sexual violence is driven by physical needs or that violent and abusive men are always angry) and make it easier for women to identify violence so they can take a stand against it. We wanted our book to be like a warm presence – a sister reaching out her hand to other sisters – to help us all rediscover the courage we need to prioritise our own safety and well-being.

We know that the violence we face as women doesn't only take place in Afghanistan, but also impacts women in the diaspora. We know that in the deep corners of our communities around the world, women continue to face abuse and struggle with familial, cultural, legal and economic barriers to seeking safety and freedom. And even when they have overcome those barriers, we know that the trauma of emotional abuse often makes it hard for survivors to start over.

You Are Not Alone is a part of a vast amount of activism centred on ending violence against women in Afghanistan. It is encouraging to see that women and our allies are reporting violence against women more than ever before and that the legal system is evolving to respond to women's needs. We are far from achieving a legal and justice system that protects and prevents violence against women, but in recent years, because of the courage of survivors seeking justice, the path to freedom has become slightly easier.

This work is important because even today, the vast majority of Afghan women face violence at home and the most brutal forms of violence, rape, physical violence and forced marriage are inflicted on them based on the decisions of their male family members.

While I have focused most of my work on Afghanistan, the place that I've called home for the majority of my life, we all know that violence against women is a global issue. It harms all women and girls, even if they are not directly impacted by it, but it also hurts everyone else. Violence against women prevents us, as a human race, from having genuine trusting relationships. It prevents us from being our most free, our most sincere selves.

It traps women in a psychological minefield of constantly making decisions based on the best ways to protect themselves from rape and violence, whether it is by carrying our keys between our fingers when we walk home or by fearing men we don't know when we walk by them on a desolate street. But it also robs men of their humanity, of the opportunity to hear women's stories and learn about our fears and dreams and capabilities. It creates a barrier that makes it hard for us to connect as people. It prevents us from seeing who we are as whole human beings.

This is why men have a moral duty to help end violence against women. They are also frequently in a higher position of power, so they have more influence when it comes to speaking out against violence. The role of men, in Afghanistan and around the world, is to bring about equality first at their own homes. They need to be questioning their families' harmful practices and traditions, and advocate for the rights of the women in their lives.

Men who claim to love us have a responsibility to change the devastating realities facing our societies. A big part of that is first and foremost acknowledging that violence against women is an issue and working towards redefining masculinity and gender roles to make violence unacceptable.

It takes every single one of us and our silence to sustain the structures that protect abusers and allow violence to continue. It will take every one of us to end it.

Mawloda Tamana Nazari: The struggle for women's health

Mawloda Tamana Nazari studied Political Science at university and works within the government sector in Afghanistan. She is a ministry secretary for the Minister of Education. Mawloda is dedicated to human rights and has worked as an executive director for an organisation called Helping Hands for Women.

During the past three decades, Afghanistan has been in a morass; the civil war may have passed, but it caused a great deal of damage and negative effects on Afghan society, especially in women's lives. The Taliban government, which ruled for five years in Afghanistan, was the darkest age for women. They couldn't go anywhere alone, they couldn't raise their voices and couldn't go outside without their family members, even for healthcare and treatment. The barriers to their lives held women back from being able to access facilities, especially for health.

There is still insufficient health provision for women in Afghanistan. We can see some facilities in the capital, Kabul, but when you observe the provinces, there are not the same services. Women living in Kabul today can get access to hospitals and clinics, but these are not available for those living in the countryside. There are two reasons for this: on the one hand, the Afghan government is not showing any attempt to provide easy access to healthcare for women; and on the other, a significant number of districts are under Taliban control (about 15 per cent of the total, according to the January 2019 report from the Special Inspector General for Afghanistan Reconstruction, or SIGAR) and they do not allow clinics and hospitals for women.

A public survey has shown that even in the capital there are not enough psychotherapy clinics to treat women. Women are suffering from anxiety, depression, stress and schizophrenia, but most don't even know about psychic disorders and mental illness. Afghans' suffering is great. One of the biggest issues for women is the high cost of medicine. In some of the provinces, drugs are not available and so they tackle their troubles with homemade medicine.

♀

The situation of women in Afghanistan is changing, but these testimonies are witness to the fact that women's access to public and private spaces, safety and security, and basic healthcare are still challenged on a daily basis. With a maturing female population comes an increasing need to enhance awareness and education about menopause to ensure the health of women at all layers of society. It is hoped that by giving voice to the issues women are facing now in Afghanistan, the time will come when such help is at hand.

17

Nursing the Menopause

2020 is the International Year of the Nurse and Midwife; in honour of this, the Australian Nursing and Midwifery Federation brings together voices from across its membership to reflect on their own and their patients' experiences of menopause, including reflections on the cultural needs of the Aboriginal community.

This year, 2020, has been designated by the World Health Organization (WHO) as the International Year of the Nurse and Midwife. The Australian Nursing and Midwifery Federation (ANMF) represents more than 285,000 nurses, midwives and carers across Australia. Our members work in the public and private health, aged care and disability sectors across a wide variety of urban, rural and remote locations. We work with them to improve their ability to deliver safe and best practice care in each and every one of these settings, fulfil their professional goals and achieve a healthy work–life balance. The ANMF is both a trade union and a professional organisation, with eight state and territory branches. These branches offer members support, industrial representation, educational opportunities through forums and conferences, professional and career development. They also campaign for improvements to wages and conditions and promote the nursing and midwifery roles in the provision of all health services.

Women comprise 89 per cent of ANMF workforce; nursing and midwifery is a predominantly female profession. Our members are uniquely placed to speak on menopause, as not only will many personally face menopause during their careers, but they also carry the responsibility of caring for those experiencing it. Nurses and midwives are well positioned with expert professional knowledge of both the physical and psychological symptoms alongside a commitment to improving health outcomes for women. But they too deserve support during the menopausal years. Sharing stories, support and connections with friends, family and peers, along with access to universal healthcare, positive work environments and professional supports, are all crucial during this time. We need to encourage an environment where woman can feel safe and supported in sharing their individual experiences of menopause.

Anita Stirling: 'I know that if I'm tired, I need to sleep'

Anita is a nurse in rural Victoria, working in the Emergency Department, and has been in nursing for eighteen years. She entered perimenopause at the age of 36.

I'm 38 and live in a small country town in regional Victoria with a population of around 1,500. I work in Emergency in a nearby city, about 65 kilometres away. I have a graduate certificate in critical care and I am also a paramedic. I've been a nurse since December 2002 and went to university straight from school. Nursing was my first preference for study, and I'm not really sure what drew me to it. My mum and my aunt are both nurses, as well as two of my older cousins. I think it's just in the blood! I'm married and have been for ten wonderful years. My husband and I have three gorgeous children between the ages of 4 and 9.

Highs and lows of my nursing job? I love that every day is different. I help people when they are at their most vulnerable, from paediatrics through to people in their last moments of life, and I work with a great team, from nursing staff to medical. I love the teamwork we have in the Emergency

Department between the medical and nursing team. The lows are the unexpected deaths from trauma. Also, not being able to help someone as much as you would like, as I'm time poor, stretched to the limit with other patients, and I just don't have the time I need.

Perimenopause! Oh what fun … I thought for a long time I was just going crazy. I was exhausted after the birth of our third child. I had anxiety, insomnia, exhaustion, hair falling out, hot flushes. At the time I put it down to hormones and 'being busy' – I had three children under 5! I went and saw my gynaecologist when I started flooding through both tampons and pads at the same time. My period started coming every two weeks, then not for five, then again after a week. She was great – I had the full work-up for everything under the sun (from thyroid to liver function tests, also known as LFTs) to make sure nothing sinister was going on. We sat down and had a very serious chat about my hormone levels being 'off' and how she thought I was going into menopause – and was I planning on having more children? I was 36 years old.

We had decided we would be content with our three, but it was still quite shattering having that decision taken away from me. I ended up having a D&C (dilation and curettage), which removes tissue inside the uterus, and a Mirena (a type of hormonal intrauterine device, or IUD) inserted – which was life-changing! The hot flushes and irregular heavy bleeding stopped. But I developed the most terrible burning pain when I was intimate with my husband – picture feeling the need to shove a Zooper Dooper ice block up your vagina to cool things down – so almost all intimacy stopped. I ended up going back to my gynaecologist who started me on pessaries, which have worked well to stop the pain and discomfort.

At work, though, I'm far more tired than I think I've ever been. I'm more cranky – so very irritable and angry over the smallest, most insignificant things. And that annoys me – so then I get more cranky! So I feel I'm not as professional as I was. The shift work is hard. Night shifts now knock me for six, and I never used to mind them. I haven't really spoken with work colleagues about it. People tend to not believe you if you say you are going through menopause. When I did need to take time off for the D&C and my sick certificate was from a gynaecologist, my boss presumed I was pregnant again. That was an awkward conversation, when I scored a 'congratulations'!

I think being someone who cares for everyone else we are great at recognising the *need* to care more for ourselves – we tell the carers of our patients this all the time; we refer them to social work so they have someone to talk to and discuss respite. But we are atrocious at actually looking after ourselves and put ourselves a lot lower in the priority scales. I think that, being a nurse, I was less scared of an IUD and the need for it, and had a better understanding of the hormones in the pessaries and the risk factors for breast cancer, because of my medical knowledge. So I think I went in with blinkers on but educated myself fairly quickly.

As a result of perimenopause, I've learned to listen to my body more. My children are still young, and I know that if I'm tired, I need to sleep. It doesn't matter if I climb into bed at half past seven when the kids go down. It's OK to say no to an overtime shift. I'm better with turning down roster requests and short shift changes (finishing at 10 p.m. and then back again at 7 a.m. the next morning). I'm more fatigue aware – especially as I need to drive up to an hour after work, and I'm also a paramedic. I eat more veggies and I started walking a while ago. I'm not fit, but I'm moving more. I've cut right back on my wine consumption – although I may have offset this with my coffee consumption, if I'm honest! I also make time now to read a book or have downtime in the evenings more than I ever did.

Sema Mustafa: 'As a nurse, I do feel more prepared'

For **Sema**, the lack of information about women's health when she was growing up was one of the reasons she entered nursing. Now 40, she lives in Sydney and specialises in rehabilitation.

I've been a registered nurse for six years and work in a rehabilitation hospital, where I see a range of patients, including those recovering from an amputation, stroke or knee operation. I came to nursing due to the lack of conversation about adolescence and how your body was going to change, and the lack of information about menstruation. When I got my period, my mother wasn't open about how it was normal or what the process was, or anything like that. Trying to explore that information through friends or other children my age, I soon found out that I wasn't getting all the facts. I remember jumping on the trampoline and then running inside in a panic and opening the bathroom door where my mum was, shouting, 'Mum!' and she just threw me a clean pair of underwear, slapped down a pad and said, 'This is what you do ...' and walked out. I felt so confused and her reaction then impacted on the way I felt about it. I didn't really know what a period was, I guess, because she never made it obvious that she had her period; she never left any pads or tampons lying around, she never left any evidence to get me thinking about that.

So, I became interested in becoming a nurse and knowing more about the body and being open about those discussions. I now come into work and ask someone about their bowel motion and that's a normal conversation to have with your patient, but that's not a topic that I'd discuss with my mum! I started out as a nursing assistant in a nursing home and I have fond memories about helping all those people there. Because they had dementia, they didn't really remember who I was, and I liked that I could just help them and it didn't matter who I was – it just felt good to me. After school, my mum steered me away from doing my registered nursing degree because she felt it wasn't going to be a suitable profession for me. She said: 'No, no, do dental nursing – it's more office hours and it's a bit cleaner'. So I took on her advice, being a good Turkish girl. But once I got married and had my third child, I expressed to my husband how much I wanted to go back and do my degree and he supported me through that, and so did my mum in the end.

The highlight is seeing someone go home and knowing that they are going to be OK, that they've achieved the goals they wanted with regard to the activities of daily living. The hardest part is when that doesn't happen – when they get sent back to the Emergency Department because of an infection or something else that's really hindered their healing. That and the shift work.

I'm currently 40 and perimenopause is something in the future for me. Doing this interview has given me the confidence to speak to Mum about her menopause, and I feel really grateful for that. I asked her what age she was when her periods started changing, and I feel like she may now take me a bit more seriously because I am older and because I am a nurse. I think she realises that is a normal part of conversation for us to be able to ask these awkward questions. Although, to be honest, I couldn't actually ask her face to face – I called her on the phone as I just didn't have the guts to sit down and have a coffee and ask her and look her in the eye about this, because it wasn't a subject that we spoke about.

She didn't get into menopause until she was 56, so I'm hoping that I will follow that trend and not get into menopause at 40 or in my early forties. Looking back, though, I remember visiting her and it being a cold day, and she had a light sweat on her face and she was fanning herself. She just said she didn't feel herself that day, but she didn't explain anything. She didn't say anything like, 'Oh my periods are starting to change,' and she didn't want to have a discussion about anything. But I do look back and think: 'Oh my God, that was *that*.'

I definitely think that being Turkish did play a big role in the way my mother was brought up, and in her thinking and what she's now passing on to me. She grew up with five sisters and four brothers, and at that time those things weren't spoken up about; sexuality wasn't spoken about. Your periods, or when boys ejaculate at a young age, none of that was discussed – it was all very hidden and hush-hush. I don't even know if she spoke about it with her sisters. I definitely know that even farting was like, 'Shush!' Everything was so private. I never saw her naked body. If we accidentally walked in on her, she screamed her head off, as though it was so wrong of us to have done that without knocking. I really do feel like those values and the way that she thought were a big part of her growing up and the way that her mother taught her to be.

However, I have to say that it stops there, with me. I don't want that for my children and, in fact, I worry about them getting the wrong information from children of their age and I'm so open, even with my boys, about periods and whatnot. I want them to be able to discuss it with me and I want them to be able to trust that they're going to get the right information from me about hormones and the changes that they're going to go through and not go seeking that information on the internet or from their mates.

My sister-in-law is a registered nurse and she went through 'the change', as she called it, a couple of years ago, and her discussion about it and her being open about her symptoms and how she was feeling about it was a real help to me. She'd tell me about her hot flushes and how they came out of nowhere, and how she just didn't feel great – that she didn't feel feminine enough any more, or her not having any natural vaginal lubrication any more, and these topics were really interesting to me, as I'd really felt in the dark and hadn't had that discussion with anyone before. Having that conversation with her has really enlightened me with regard to what to expect.

Also, as a nurse, I do feel more prepared and feel like I have a more positive attitude. Nursing allows you to look at both sides of the coin. You can look at HRT or the natural remedies that are out there and that gives you a broader choice, so you can weigh up and decide which way you want to go. I don't really have that fear of going through menopause or premenopause. I feel quite positive about it – I feel like it's something we're all going to go through. It's inevitable and I feel like you've still got to just work with it.

I think that this book is wonderful. Being open and educated and honest, and not being shy about these sorts of discussions, is such a positive move forward for everybody and every culture. The UK, as Australia, is a multicultural country and these taboos are slowly lifting, and I definitely think we're moving forward in a positive way.

Elaine Blower: 'I am now being much kinder to myself'

A nurse for 30 years, **Elaine** is an aged care assessor. Debilitating menopause symptoms have meant that she has needed to take unpaid leave from work, for the sake of her own health.

Nursing has been such a rewarding career. I was drawn to the caring aspect of the work and love to go the 'extra mile' to make my clients' experiences as holistic as possible. I started out as a ward help in a nursing home and enjoyed working with the elderly. I enrolled to complete a Division 2 registered nurse course and then gained entry to university to complete my Division 1 nursing degree. I worked on mainly surgical wards, then branched out into community care co-ordination. I also completed a graduate diploma of applied gerontology, gaining an award for my high grades.

I am married with two adult children, both of whom have left home this year; my parents are both elderly. I live in a country town and work 20 minutes away in a large city. I recently changed roles at work and commenced working for another programme, working with elderly people mainly in their own homes.

Highs of my work have been feeling like I can help and reassure people in their time of need. I have learned so much in my thirty years of nursing and never stop learning about the 'human condition'. Lows would be witnessing so much human suffering. I have been present when patients have been told of their terminal prognosis, I have nursed people with debilitating and chronic conditions, I have seen first hand the chaos of addiction and mental illness, and I have been subject to physical and verbal abuse from clients and their families. Nursing is not for the faint-hearted!

I think my most debilitating menopausal symptoms started after taking on my new role at work. I found learning a whole new system of doing things challenging and getting to know new colleagues took a lot of energy. My concentration and ability to absorb new information was declining and I felt the typical 'brain fog' associated with menopause but didn't really twig that that was it, I just thought I was tired.

I started having a lot of trouble sleeping and woke each morning with a feeling of dread. My body ached from the top of my head to the tip of my toes. I was plagued by constant ruminating each night. All of this impacted my confidence. At home the mood swings were horrendous. I felt irritable and aggressive towards my husband and was very short and sharp with the rest of my family. I have also experienced weight gain, urinary frequency, headaches, dry skin and eyes, and extreme fatigue. A few hot flushes but not many really.

I felt so unwell I went to my GP and she prescribed me HRT. I started on oestrogen gel and progesterone tablets. The hormones improved some symptoms but after a few months my period returned and lasted for three weeks. My GP instructed me to take the hormones sequentially, which was fiddly to manage, then I stopped taking it completely.

I was referred to a menopause specialist clinic in Melbourne but could not bring myself to commute the distance required to attend. I felt my GP was sympathetic but not confident treating menopause-related issues. I have also tried the contraceptive pill and hormone replacement patches unsuccessfully.

Many of my work colleagues are of similar age to me so have been through or are going through menopause themselves. We have had conversations regarding menopause symptoms in the tea room, but mostly in a joking way. I have deeper relationships with some colleagues where I have felt able to discuss my most difficult symptoms openly and not feel judged. Some of us 'compare notes' but no two of us has the same experience.

I have felt misunderstood at work at times. I find some women report what a breeze it was for them when they went through menopause and how it's a natural event in a woman's life. Sometimes women are each other's worst enemy. Currently I am on a leave of absence from work. I just couldn't continue the way I felt. Because I have used up my annual leave trying to feel better, most of my leave will be unpaid now. I have not told many people why I am not able to work as I feel I may be stigmatised. My medical certificate says I have a medical condition.

Being a nurse has helped me to understand the reasons for and the treatment of menopause, but I admit I was totally unprepared for the way it has impacted me. I was one of those people that used to joke and say, 'I can't wait until I hit menopause.' The older ladies used to look knowingly at each other and roll their eyes – now I know why!

Now I am ensuring I rest. I have taken up mindfulness meditation and regular Bowen Therapy or massage. (Bowen Therapy was founded in Australia and involves a series of moves on soft tissue to stimulate the body's self-healing mechanisms.) I have given up coffee and alcohol, am eating a Mediterranean diet with limited processed foods, exercising, and spending time with friends that 'fill my bucket'. I find all of these things help but I am a long way from well as I type. I am seeing a psychologist regularly and she has diagnosed me with burnout. I guess being in a career that involves caring, and having children, elderly parents and a husband, you put yourself last on the list of priorities. I am now being much kinder to myself, allowing myself to feel emotions and get them out. I have done a lot of crying but it has been cathartic.

Final thoughts would be that I think there should be an option at work to take 'menopause leave', just like you would take maternity leave. Maybe not all women would require it but it would be nice to have as an option. All people should be better educated about menopause and made aware that menopause is not just hot flushes, it can really impact on a woman's health and self-esteem. Women should try to be more supportive of other women, understanding that everyone's experience of menopause is different. We will all go through it at some time if we live long enough, so let's all support each other.

Faye Clarke: 'We don't mess with our aged women'

Faye Clarke, in her mid-fifties, has been in nursing for sixteen years and works at the Ballarat and District Aboriginal Collective as a diabetes nurse educator. Her cultural heritage is as a Muandik woman and for four years she has been an advisor to the ANMF Reconciliation Action Plan Working Group.

I have always had an interest in working in one of the 'helping professions'. At the age of 36, recently separated and a single parent of three children, living on a pension, I decided, with my youngest starting school, it was time for me to gain a career. I have been nursing since 2004, sixteen years now, and have been working in Aboriginal health for twelve of those years. The opportunity arose to study diabetes education in a course that was designed for First Nations health workers, so that was my entry point in 2012 into the diabetes nursing and education that I do now. My father had diabetes and died aged 41 from complications, so I was well aware of the significant impact of diabetes and wanted to make a difference in the Aboriginal community.

I work now at the Ballarat and District Aboriginal Cooperative, in the city of Ballarat in Victoria. My main source of enjoyment in my work is in meeting people, developing a rapport with them and working together to create positive change in their life to help manage the condition. My favourite times are those teaching moments when 'the penny drops' and people understand how the information relates to them personally. My lows are the frustrations of dealing with a system (Medicare) that limits or dictates how I can operate. Free medical care is an absolute imperative for our community, so I am not against Medicare – it's just the limitations I find frustrating. At the end of the day, the clients can't work with a 'colonised' system, so it's hard to bridge the gap sometimes.

In Australia, we have over 250 different Aboriginal and Torres Strait Islander countries. I am sensitive to the fact that my own personal experience will differ from that of many other Aboriginal people in the country. My maternal grandmother, from whom my Aboriginality comes, was estranged from her mother at the age of 16. My non-Aboriginal paternal grandmother was fostered many times, after the untimely death of her mother when she was a baby. I grew up in a predominantly white community despite the Aboriginal family around me. This has undoubtedly influenced my knowledge and understanding. In addition, I am a well-educated Aboriginal woman, which is not the typical experience for most.

I am in my mid-fifties and had a hysterectomy in 2008 at the age of 44, though my ovaries were left in situ. Initially I didn't notice much change, but feel like I could still sense the ups and downs of my hormonal and mood changes. PMS had been a significant feature of my life and I still experienced breast tenderness and changes to my moods, appetite and energy that I had commonly associated with PMS. Over time, however, I started to notice a decline in those and a ramping up of things like hot flushes, night sweats and insomnia. In more recent times I have noticed vaginal dryness and my partner thinks I've become more irritable. I think I have become less tolerant of things that irritate me, both at home and at work. I'm not sure if it is menopause, but when I find there are issues at work, for example around cultural safety, I am more likely to express it.

At home, bed and sleep is a battle ground, with not getting good-quality sleep and this impacting on the energy I have each day. Some days I accept I am tired and don't try to achieve too much at home. Work is a different story, in that I always work hard there, no matter how tired.

The most common symptom I hear about in my role as a nurse and in the community is hot flushes. This is something we bond and laugh about. For the most part my experience is that it is discussed in private with the GP, if the woman is comfortable to bring it up. My understanding is that women don't talk about it much. It is kept to themselves. We don't often get a chance to bring women of menopausal age together in a closed setting, so they don't get a chance to express themselves, but my guess is that women would discuss it in their peer groups. Women's and men's business is still a thing in our community so women would want other women to hear them. They may discuss issues with their partners, but it would depend how supportive their partner was and it is almost never discussed publicly.

My main influences around issues of womanhood were my mother and maternal grandmother. Both women, as did I, had hysterectomies in our middle age. Not much was mentioned to me as a child and in my menopause my mother has passed. It is not a subject that comes up with my grandmother. She has always been fairly quiet about these things unless the topic comes up and she feels free to talk. Hot flushes are acknowledged, but not much else. My cultural heritage is as a Muandik woman, and ageing is something that is well respected in our community, with importance given to wisdom. We don't mess with our aged women but respectfully wait until you have been spoken to.

The impact of colonisation has been difficult in that generational conversations have been interfered with and the knowledge of times past has been interrupted. This has a big impact on future generations of women.

I have been fortunate to work with some great female GPs over the years. They have been a font of knowledge for women in our community. Generally, clients seek advice individually from them but on two occasions that I recall we had the GPs speak at women's health promotion days and I have learned a lot from those about menopause and how to manage this time in your life. In particular I recall being taught it is just a cycle of life and to revere and respect that time where life is freer. It was a very positive outlook.

For women in my community, I find that many have had a limited understanding of menopause and of how your body works. This applies to diabetes as well, in that we need to teach people what is actually going on. For most they have not been privy to conversations about menopause, much like me, so they are just as naïve. Our mothers and grandmothers may have referred to it as 'the change of life', but that just kept it all the more a mystery. I never bothered to ask what the change was, except for knowing it was the end of the dreaded monthlies: nothing to grieve there.

As a nurse, I might be aware of the need to care for myself, but find it difficult to do. I am a full-time worker with three adult children, two grandchildren, five nieces and nephews who are without a parent, their eight children, a grandmother and the occasional aunt, uncle or cousin with something that needs following up. I try to manage our cohort of patients with diabetes and a multitude of clients with complex needs. There is not a lot of time for myself, as my partner would attest.

When I checked in on what was happening locally in terms of support for women experiencing issues with menopause, all the women in my workplace were silent. However, the peak body for Aboriginal health in Australia is working on ways to open up the conversation. I am looking forward to their innovative ways to engage women in a dialogue about menopause – we should talk more about it, so we don't have to feel so alone in our symptoms.

18

Demystifying the Menopause: The Research, Medicine and Education We All Need

Dr Wen Shen, Assistant Professor in the Johns Hopkins Medicine Department of Gynaecology and Obstetrics, and Dr Christine Ekechi, Consultant Obstetrician and Gynaecologist at Imperial Healthcare NHS Trust, share their specialist expertise in treating women throughout their lives and their passionate advocacy for better menopause health education. These views were given during two separate interviews and have been brought together here to show the issues facing women's healthcare practice in both the US and UK.

Getting into gynaecology

Dr Wen Shen

I've always been told by my mother that I am here because she had amazing obstetrical care. My parents went to Taiwan from mainland China in the 1950s. Both my older sisters were born in mainland China; I was the only one of three babies born on Taiwan to survive childbirth. Back then, Taiwan still had very poor medical care, so my mother said she was awfully lucky to have been taken care of by probably the only qualified obstetrician in Taiwan at that time. I was my mother's easiest birth, even though I weighed 8lb. Apparently, all the nurses in the hospital came running over to look at me, because no one had ever seen such a big, fat baby before – at that point, most Chinese babies were only about 5lb. My mother attributed her easy birth to this amazing woman who was her obstetrician, so that put a very positive light on women obstetricians for me since early childhood. My mother herself was an amazingly strong woman. She passed away in 2014, but to this day, when we talk about her, my husband talks about everything she'd accomplished. She helped my father move from mainland China to Taiwan, then to Brazil, and eventually we came to the US. And through it all, as my father always said, she was his backbone, and she held the family together. She was an inspirational mother figure. She made me want to work with women and be an obstetrician to help women.

I spent the first twenty years of my medical career in general obstetrics and gynaecology (OB-GYN) and then I specialised in gynaecology only, and specifically, in menopause medicine. Menopause called to me because during those first twenty years, I took care of a lot of menopausal women who came to me with symptoms and problems. When I first started practice right after my residency, I realised I knew nothing about menopause because we weren't really taught it. We had a lot of training in obstetrics, so I felt remarkably capable in obstetrics, even very complicated high-risk obstetrics. I also felt highly capable in general gynaecology. But when it came to patients with menopause issues, I was left virtually clueless. Menopause medicine was in its infancy and we were not trained during residency. I started reading as much as I could on my own. I also had very well-educated patients, who did a lot of research, and who knew more than I did. So, I learned from them. I joined an organisation in the US called the North American Menopause Society (NAMS) and I credit them for educating me and instilling in me a passion for menopause medicine. I can't help but wonder if my mother's quality of life in her last decades could have been improved by what we know now.

When my children became more self-sufficient, I started thinking about going back to Johns Hopkins to see what they were doing about menopause. This was back in 2005 and Hopkins still wasn't teaching menopause. So, I went to the chairman of the department, Dr Fox, and I have to give him credit, because I had no additional training outside of my basic OB-GYN training; I did not do a fellowship. I said, 'I want to do this. I want to focus on menopause. Will you take me in as faculty, so that I can start teaching the residents?' And to my utter delight and surprise he said yes.

Dr Christine Ekechi

I was the classic 1980s child of Nigerian parents, for whom medicine is seen as one or the *only* profession to go into. Parents tend to be very limited in their discussions with their children about professions and, to be honest, I wanted to please my dad. And as a young child you want to help people, you just have no idea of what it actually means to be a doctor. When I went to medical school, OB-GYN was not at the top of my list. Initially I wanted to be a general surgeon, but when I started early training I realised that it wasn't really for me. Back then, general surgery wasn't really accommodating for women, so it was suggested that I try OB-GYN. I joined a team that was very open and welcoming, and I fell in love with it straight away. Part of it was this ability to have an impact that then resulted in something positive, which was new life on the obstetrics side, and also being able to perform surgeries to improve women's health where needed, on the gynaecology side. As a specialism, it provided a wealth of opportunities – whether I decided to go and specialise in fertility, or scan, identify and treat gynaecological cancers, or, indeed, obstetrics.

It also very much fulfilled my other interests in travelling. I got into public health and OB-GYN in lower-income settings, looking at the differences in the health experiences of women outside the UK. I spent a lot of time doing work around this in my extra time.

Now my time is split between NHS work, private work and advocacy. In my clinical work, I'm dual-trained as an obstetrician and gynaecologist, with a specialist interest in early pregnancy, where I see women who present anywhere on their life-health arc. It might be that they come along very early in pregnancy and I perform scans to confirm that the pregnancy is developing well, or I may see them in the antenatal period to ensure we achieve a good outcome for the mother and baby, or on the labour ward when they may come to deliver. I may also see women in the postnatal period or indeed if women present with gynaecological problems, or later in life during the menopause. My job really encompasses treating women throughout their life arc. That's one of the other great things about OB-GYN – you are really seeing women through all stages and not just at particular snapshots in their lives.

Menopause in medical practice

Dr Wen Shen

The first, most common symptom that I see in my clinic is abnormal uterine bleeding. For women going through the menopause transition, and for women who are postmenopausal, the abnormal bleeding can be quite scary. My role is to reassure and thoroughly evaluate them, and then administer the proper treatment. The second most common symptom is hot flushes. For some women, this can be so severe that their quality of life is completely ruined. Some women have palpitations and heart-racing that almost feels like a panic attack associated with the hot flushes. In addition, they think they're having a heart attack and have a sense of doom. It's hard to work when they are experiencing such debilitating symptoms. Some women have these extreme hot flushes seven or more times a day. How can they function at work? These symptoms will also obviously influence their relationship with their families. Often these flushes also happen at night, so women are being awakened several times a night, and in the most severe cases they literally have to get up and change their sleepwear and their bedsheets, because they're soaked. If this happens even once a night it disrupts sleep, and for some women it happens several times in the night. These women become sleep deprived, which affects their cognition and mood as well as health. We know that sleep deprivation can in the long term lead to heart disease, early onset dementia, weight gain, and many other bad health consequences. So, having hot flushes and night sweats are no laughing matter. I know that it's been a source of jokes in the past, but we now know of the medical ramifications of these hot flushes.

Then the next most common issue is vaginal symptoms which can include vaginal dryness and painful intercourse. These can also be extremely distressing, because, before we even talk about sex, the dryness and the discomfort can make the simple act of urination painful because it burns the skin. Many of these symptoms can be traced back to the oestrogen and progesterone receptors. Women have oestrogen and progesterone receptors on practically every organ of the body. The pelvic floor, the vaginal skin, the vulvar skin and the bladder are all very oestrogen-rich areas. When a woman becomes postmenopausal, the lack of oestrogen causes the skin in all these areas to become very thin. Premenopause, the skin of a woman's vagina is usually many cell layers deep. On vaginal exam of a premenopausal woman, her vagina is a ruddy pink colour with lots of folds, which are called rugae. This thickness of the skin, the folds in the vagina and also the mucus production from the glands allow a woman's vagina to remain healthy and be comfortable, as well as allowing it to stretch when she's having intercourse or giving birth to a baby. Postmenopausally, the skin in the vagina is very thin, it's a single cell layer and the skin appears pale pink, maybe even white, and there are no folds in it. Even using a very small paediatric speculum can cause discomfort to some patients. The skin on the outside, on the vulva, likewise becomes thin, and has a crêpey appearance. These atrophic skin changes also occur in the bladder. Hence the bladder can't stretch and it becomes much more sensitive to even the smallest amount of urine and so a lot of women will have issues with urgent incontinence or having to get up multiple times a night to empty their bladder.

Other common symptoms include hair loss, weight gain and loss of libido. These symptoms tend to be less amenable to hormone therapy because they have multiple contributing factors. The loss of ovarian hormones definitely contributes to hair loss, but there are many other reasons for hair loss as women age. Similarly with weight gain and libido. Menopause can also be a time of great stress for a lot of women, because of family matters, because of being the sandwich generation, because of work, and all of this contributes to stress. It is also the time when a lot of women start developing metabolic syndrome, with diabetes, high blood pressure and high cholesterol. Beyond the physical symptoms of menopause, there are many mental symptoms that patients will experience, such as brain fog, mood swings and depression, which can be due to menopausal hormone changes. Throughout their lives, women have times of hormonal vulnerability: at puberty (anybody with a daughter between the ages of 9 and 16 will understand this), during pregnancy and at menopause. These are very distinctive times of hormonal variability, changes and instability. Women are much more vulnerable to mood issues during these stages. Depression has been shown to be an aspect for some women going through the perimenopause – anxiety too. These may be separate issues, but they definitely feed into each other. Irritability is also very common. Many of my patients say things like, 'my husband's ready to walk out', 'my kids think I'm the meanest mom' and 'I just screamed at my boss'. These reactions occur because there are oestrogen receptors all over the brain too, and oestrogen helps with moods, depression and brain fog. Oestrogen also helps with neuronal connections, and its activity has been shown in specific parts of the brain that process memory, multitasking and language. As a woman goes through perimenopause, her hormone levels vary greatly. Once a woman is postmenopausal that variation diminishes. One of my colleagues likened the menopause transition to flying over the Rockies. What she meant was that when one flies across the US from the East Coast to the West Coast, one flies over the Rocky Mountains, where there's often atmospheric turbulence. But once over the Pacific, the turbulence usually calms down. Once a woman gets through the menopause transition, everything tends to calm down.

There are other medical conditions that are vital for a woman to understand which are not widely known by women to be associated with the menopause, but that are profoundly influenced by the loss of ovarian hormones. Cardiovascular disease is the primary killer of women after 65. A patient can be horribly symptomatic with menopause, but yet she is scared to go on hormones because her mother had breast cancer at the age of 80. While cancer is terrifying and life altering, breast cancer is pretty far down on the list of causes of mortality for women after the age of 65, while cardiovascular disease is right up there as number one. All through a woman's reproductive years oestrogen protects her heart, as well as her bones, brain and other organs. But once a woman becomes postmenopausal, the loss of oestrogen increases her risk of cardiovascular disease, and there are studies that confirm the benefit of oestrogen on heart health, especially for young women with premature menopause.

Osteoporosis is another big issue because people are not aware of how dangerous osteoporosis is. People think, 'Oh, I'll get more stooped, maybe I'll get shorter.' But the risk is in fragility fractures, and the fact is that about 50 per cent of all women will get osteoporosis-related fractures. Once a woman has a fragility fracture, she doesn't just bounce back from it. It's not like breaking a bone skiing in her twenties – put a cast on it and six weeks later, she is back on the slopes. With fragility fractures, a large percentage of women – as high as 80 per cent – never get back to their previous lifestyle. They lose their independence and mobility, and their body habits change. They are immobilised and depression sets in. It's this chain reaction that happens with osteoporosis that I think the general public is not aware of. The number one thing on everybody's mind is cancer and everybody knows mostly what they need to do to avoid cancers. But osteoporosis is so important and with early diagnosis, proper lifestyle and medications as needed, one can go a long way towards preventing it. Genetics is an important factor after menopause. If a woman has a maternal history of osteoporosis, she needs to be proactive, starting with her menopause transition.

Dr Christine Ekechi

A lot of the women I see are understandably anxious about the symptoms that they're experiencing and aren't sure whether to attribute them to the approaching menopause or menopause itself. They are also very much worried that the impact of the symptoms they are experiencing currently will be long term and detrimental to their quality of life going forward. These symptoms tend to be the headline ones that are most often mentioned, but of course menopausal symptoms may manifest in a number of ways. This may include concerns about difficulty in maintaining concentration at work and the impact this may have on their productivity, difficulty in sleeping and changes to their libido – that's a very common presentation – as well as vaginal dryness. Sometimes it's a case of a woman saying, 'I just don't feel right' and not being able to pin it down using medical lexicon, but rather, a feeling.

Endometriosis is also one of the most common reasons why people will present in gynaecology clinics. Often women present with painful periods, which is a common sign of endometriosis. The difficulty with endometriosis is that there are no specific outward signs, other than pain (and pain is subjective), so it can be very difficult to achieve a diagnosis in a timely manner and for a long time the only way to definitely confirm a diagnosis was with surgery. This surgery takes the form of a laparoscopy to see the endometriotic deposits, but even then, there isn't a very good correlation between the degree of pain a woman reports and the degree of endometriosis that we find. For example, we might find people with severe endometriosis clinically, who may have minimal symptoms, or conversely you can have a woman who presents with lots of pain and a diagnostic laparoscopy demonstrates minimal endometriosis. What we don't want to do is a laparoscopy for everybody, because a laparoscopy in itself is an operation that carries risk. Therefore, where a woman gives a history that is highly indicative of endometriosis, we may commence a treatment course as a trial of treatment. Women with endometriosis will normally respond to this treatment. Currently, the best treatments we have to hand are hormonal treatments, but we also know that lifestyle measures can also significantly improve the symptoms that a woman may experience.

Endometriosis at its worst can be very debilitating and there are those infrequent cases where very severe disease may require a hysterectomy. In these situations and more broadly, it's important to consider the psychological impact of any gynaecological condition on a person. These impacts can be profound, because for a long time society has very much defined what it means to be a woman and this definition centres around a woman's body and her gynaecological organs. Women have often internalised these ideas such that difficulties with gynaecological conditions are viewed as negatively impinging on 'womanhood'. Additionally, society places a significant emphasis on youth, and particularly female youth and a woman's ability to reproduce. Where this role is unable to be fulfilled – be it due to a surgical cessation of periods and ovulation or the inability to have a child resulting from the surgical removal of the uterus due to a gynaecological condition, the psychological impact may be significant on the whole identity of that individual.

For women who find themselves at these crossroads where symptoms may be debilitating enough that significant treatment is required, it is important that as medical professionals we counsel them of the benefits and risks to treatment taking into account their needs as a whole. We must have a full, open and frank conversation with a woman so that she's able to make a decision that is based on what is best for her.

The research we need

Dr Wen Shen
So much needs to be researched, because until only recently most research was done on men. Now at least it's normal that research includes both men and women. Women do respond differently to diseases and medications than men. There needs to be basic research in every specialty. Definitely cardiology has improved in that regard. There is a much better understanding about female cardiology after menopause. A better understanding of postmenopause neurological and cognitive conditions

is also needed. For example, why is it that so many more women have Alzheimer's than men? There are similar questions in rheumatologic diseases like lupus, which is much more prevalent in women.

Every aspect of menopause health needs more research. The practice of medicine often occurs in silos; the right hand doesn't know what the left hand is doing, and the wheel is being reinvented in so many ways. Meanwhile, the poor woman is stuck in the middle, trying to figure out for herself which doctor she should be seeing. My vision is for an integrated form of supplying medical care for women as we age, and I think this will be the best way to give healthcare, and it will be more efficient too. Currently, there is much repetition and waste, not just the money but also waste of time for the patient. So much time is wasted when diagnoses are missed that could have been made months (or even years) ago, had the physicians spoken to each other. And this time is often spent living in pain and misery for the woman. This is something that I'm really passionate about, which is why I am setting up a Women's Wellness and Healthy Aging Program at at Hopkins. This will be for women who are 45 and above and prematurely menopausal women to obtain preventive healthy ageing care as well as integrated focused care for women who are at increased risk of illnesses.

Dr Christine Ekechi
There have been a number of articles and research that have explored gender and ethnic biases in medicine. Within gynaecology these biases exist when looking at outcomes for conditions such as endometriosis or indeed cancer.

It is important to even out any gaps in medicine where they may exist, be it a gender gap or, in this particular context, an ethnicity gap. We need to collect the data. We cannot know how deep the ocean is unless we measure. So, collecting the data is the first and most important thing to emphasise. The second is that we need to be much better at how we collect the data, especially by ethnicity. One area of research that has been particularly lacking is that around fibroids, a condition that affects a significant portion of Black and Asian women, and which can be extremely debilitating. Currently, without more research, we're no better at really understanding why certain women or certain groups have a high incidence of fibroids or why there is a prevalence of fibroids in Black and Asian women. Without this information our interventions cannot significantly progress further than existing surgical methods that we know carry a level of risk.

The menopause education we all need

Dr Wen Shen

I really can't emphasise education enough. Not just for the providers, but also the patients. To be educated about their health, about their menopause health, is the ultimate empowerment for patients, because then they know what questions to ask and what they can expect. Menopausal women need evidence-based information to be widely disseminated. They often fall prey to the overwhelming number of online mis-information sites, and questionable 'treatments', which are ineffective and maybe dangerous. Some of the older patients, after consultation with me, will say, 'If I had only known that ...' And that is a shame, because their previous doctors just didn't know. And it's no fault of the doctors, because they were never trained in it. There needs to be more awareness.

I think that we are still in the very beginning stages, but at least there is awareness now that menopause medicine is necessary. I know at Hopkins, and I think in most university programmes, internal medicine residents have an option to focus in women's health. That's a big step forward. Women's health has traditionally focused on the reproductive age group. But with the ageing of the world's population, women in industrialised countries are living a third of their lives (as much as thirty years) in postmenopause, so menopause medicine should become a public health agenda. Public policy makers need to be educated on this need to achieve optimal health for women in the post-reproductive phase of their lives.

Dr Christine Ekechi

You would think that an issue affecting 50 per cent of the population at some point in their lives, as long as they are to reach that age, would be something that we all understand well and can manage by ourselves and within the community, but that's not necessarily the case.

The first place to start is education for women. Once we are educated, we have the power of knowledge and are better able to advocate for ourselves. This includes men as well as women. We must demystify menopause – it's something that should be spoken about much more openly. We are getting there. In the past three years I've heard much more open conversations and it is positive.

There remains a fear from doctors who don't come across women with menopausal symptoms in their daily medical practice but normally all that is required is a listening ear. The large number of HRT options for women can be daunting and the information regarding risks, scary. By clearly explaining options and risks, women can make the choice that is right for them. It is important to reassure women that overall the risks remain small, but if risks outweigh the benefits for some women, there are a number of alternative treatments so that no woman has to suffer with uncomfortable menopausal symptoms.

There are also cultural issues to take into account. Some women are more vocal about issues surrounding the menopause than others and for some women from ethnic minority groups they may not be as vocal about their menopause symptoms; this may be due to cultural habits but may also be due to how symptoms are experienced and in some instances normalised, such that they do not pose a negative impact on a woman's life. The most important thing we can do is to listen and support women in the best way that we can. This will be different for each and every woman.

Dr Wen Shen is an Assistant Professor in the Department of Gynecology and Obstetrics at the Johns Hopkins University School of Medicine and the Johns Hopkins School of Nursing. She is also the Director of the Menopause Consultation Service and the Co-director of the Women's Wellness and Healthy Aging Program at Johns Hopkins. She spent the first 18 years of her medical career in general practice of OB-GYN. She returned to Johns Hopkins and joined the faculty in 2005. Since then her primary focus has been on menopause education to the medical community as well as the lay public. Dr Shen's lectures on menopause are part of the curriculum for residents, medical students, nurse doctoral candidates and public health students. She conducted the first national survey of menopause education in OB-GYN residency across the United States and established the first Johns Hopkins Menopause Medicine Curriculum and Resident Menopause Clinic. She produced the Johns Hopkins Menopause App through a grant from Pfizer, which has been downloaded internationally. She has been the recipient of teaching awards from the residents at Johns Hopkins, as well as the 2019 NAMS/ Leon Speroff Outstanding Educator Award.

Dr Christine Ekechi specialises in early pregnancy and acute gynaecology care. Using her experience in ultrasound and outpatient management of benign gynaecological conditions, her focus is on the provision of patient-focused, accessible, high-quality care convenient to the busy lifestyles that women lead. Dr Ekechi has a specialised interest in ultrasound in early pregnancy and acute gynaecology and in the hysteroscopic management of fibroids. She is also an accredited colposcopist and is an advocate for cervical screening and awareness. She has also worked with the United Nations in New York.

19

Becoming Wise Women

Lynne Franks, communications powerhouse, founder of the SEED women's empowerment network and author of the globally renowned *The SEED Handbook*, on sustainable enterprise with feminine values, champions how women can harness their innate wisdom and power as they age.

I guess I was 51 or 52 when my periods stopped. I'm 71 now, so it's a long time ago for me. My perimenopause consisted of incredibly heavy periods with a lot of pain and also fibroids, so for me menopause was a huge relief. I was in California, where I was living an outdoor life, in the sunshine every day. I was eating healthily, living healthily, doing lots of exercise. I did go and see a specialist doctor in America, who put me on to wild yam for a couple of months. Then in England I went to see a top doctor and she put me on to HRT. I started taking it for a month and then I just thought, 'This is insane, I don't know what I'm doing,' and stopped. And I didn't need anything, really.

I had hot flushes, and I can sometimes still get one if I drink wine, tea or coffee in an airless room. I controlled the symptoms as well as I could through diet. I used to go every three months to somewhere that special-ised in wheatgrass and fasting and enemas. I was also seeing a very good

Chinese acupuncturist in LA, and he said no hot food; keep away from chilli – because if you're already hot, you'll get hotter, and it's just heating up the blood the whole time. It's common sense, really. I became aware very quickly that if I avoided toxins, I would not get the worst of the symptoms. I didn't drink coffee, I didn't drink alcohol. And I changed my whole menopause experience. My recommendations are: no sugar; no dairy; cut the alcohol right down (nothing if you can get away with it); no coffee definitely; no teas; good natural supplements. Everything should be as natural as possible. Traditionally the Japanese don't even have a word for menopause; they have a different diet of fish, veggies and soya, although of course these days more are eating a Western diet of fat and sugar.

I'd also recommend yoga, meditation and dance. I, like so many women of all ages, love to dance. It's part of our DNA and yet so easy to let go of. It's a very important aspect of well-being in all the generations in my family. I've been doing Gabrielle Roth's Five Rhythms classes since I was in my early forties and it put me back in touch with my dance. In LA I'd be going to Five Rhythms classes two or three times a week alongside many other wonderful women and men also dedicated to this spiritual movement practice, which literally danced me through menopause. I also like to do a bit of boxing if I can. Anything that can get the body moving. Also connecting with nature, with the earth. I'm not a great gardener – I love my gardens but I'm not personally very good at it – but I love *being* in nature. I think it's very important. There's the whole thing about the healing hormone oxytocin, which is released particularly when you're with small children, or animals, or other women, talking in a group. That's why it helps the 'feel-good' aspect of life if you have animals: it's no coincidence that older women often have a small dog at their heels. Very healthy. And as our libido and confidence come back during menopause, it is important to have some kind of sexual activity. Orgasms are healthy and even if you are not with someone regularly, even self-love keeps the body ticking over. I had more lovers when I was in my suddenly single fifties than at any other time in my life, which was definitely good for my health.

I had got divorced at around 49, sold my business and gone to live in California. I also stopped doing my Buddhist practice at the time (although I have reconnected with it now). So, all these things happened fairly quickly. Everything was in freefall, and at the same time I had started going through my menopause. Looking back, it was perfect for me to not be living my former highly stressed life running my business in London, and to be in a beautiful, sunny place like California. I don't think menopause influenced those changes in my life; I think it's just timing. When you're around 50, that's when you take a look at life – and also when you're 30, and when you're 70 ... it doesn't stop. But 50 does seem to be a particularly important time for reflection and change. So much depends on whether you have children, if the children are still young, and if your parents are getting frail. It's about circumstance. My children were just getting old enough to leave home and travel themselves. They were in their late teens, so they were finding themselves. My life has always been subject to a huge amount of synchronicity. Perfect synchronicity. It's not about what is supposed to be, or isn't supposed to be; it just goes in that kind of flow. At that point in my life there was a synchronicity and a flow which encompassed the menopause but was not because of the menopause. It's that period in life when so many different aspects of life can go through major changes, including how we feel about ourselves, our self-confidence and our physicality.

I don't think menopause should be treated like an illness. I hate the amount of pharmaceutical drugs that are doled out for every ache and pain, and I'm not convinced that people aren't being given those drugs who don't need them. Menopause is a crucial passage of womanhood which we get through, and it's not the end of the world. We have a few upsets, we can have mood swings and depressions, but I believe we can get over all of those things if we have a basic healthy diet and the right supplements. And once we are on the other side, there is clarity and health and libido and all the lovely things in life without all those hormonal swings. Your sex life can be easier; you don't have to worry about taking the pill. This time can be about really learning to be true to yourself. It can be a healthy passage, a welcoming passage. I also think it's important to ritualise it with your women friends in celebration and ceremony.

I've been working with women and women's empowerment for the last twenty-odd years since I sold my PR business. In the early 1990s, I was asked to chair a women's radio station and through that I got involved in a lot of women's initiatives and conferences where I started to understand what was going on for so many women all over the world. I became heavily involved in the women's movement. It found me, in a way. In 1995, I put on an event called 'What Women Want' at the South Bank, which at that time was the first major UK public gathering for women on all aspects of women's lives in the modern day. It was time for women to start talking about things that currently meant a lot to them in a public forum: natural health, our power to be sustainable consumers and business owners, understanding technology, the environment, all areas of creativity including song, owning our sexuality and many other subjects. Even though 1995 doesn't seem that long ago, the world was hugely different – we were only just starting to use the internet. Wonderful Anita Roddick, founder of the Body Shop, sadly no longer with us, supported me in a lot of this. We had women learning how to go online, we had a fantastic concert with Sinéad O'Connor and Chrissie Hynde, we had nuns, a whole awareness of the sacred feminine in society. It was extraordinary; we took over the whole of the South Bank. That was August, and then the next week I went to China for the UN Women's Conference in Beijing, which was a very important experience for me, meeting so many women from different countries, cultures and backgrounds. From there I started speaking at women's events all around the world continuing to meet extraordinary women and hearing their stories.

I felt that it was coming to a point where a lot of women would leave the corporate world and start their own small businesses, particularly now they had the important access to the internet. So, when I went to live in California, apart from starting a new marketing and PR business myself, I wrote *The SEED Handbook: The Feminine Way to Create Business* – now celebrating its twenty-year anniversary. SEED is an acronym for Sustainable Enterprise and Empowerment Dynamics. It became a bestselling book all over the English-speaking world, in Germany, in Japan; it's just come out in Russian, and other countries such as Kazakhstan. SEED became a whole body of content, and a series of tools and training, that has been used as a leadership model for women in this country and others to start their own businesses. SEED has been delivered in women's prisons as well as working with The Prince's Trust, with disadvantaged young women on the streets. We had a project with the World Bank, for women producing hand knitwear; I worked in African villages. This is alongside SEED becoming a women's leadership programme for corporate boardrooms. It has had a huge impact on thousands of women all over the world and continues to develop as a global women's platform for change.

My Power of Seven women's leadership programme, based on seven traditional feminine archetypes such as Medicine Woman and Story Teller, is a recent development and is an ongoing aspect of the programmes which

I am workshopping on- and offline in workshops and retreats. Power of Seven starts with the balance and harmony of these different aspects in each of us. Then, if we form a small pod or circle of seven women to create a business or a community initiative, we can all take one of the roles or archetypes to collaborate together most effectively on creating something more powerful than when we do it on our own.

Although it's not exclusively for women, I think it is a way that women can work in small groups on a local level and create change. That's what I'm doing. I live in Wincanton, a small town in Somerset, and we're working together in a group here about creating change in our community. And then we're tying in with the bigger picture with the council and other bodies.

I've been coaching people on Power of Seven for the last two years, and we've had a few projects that have been done in Frome and some other places. The seven archetypes are also a way to help these groups continue. I've always found with women's groups that people come in with the best will, but they get busy, or their child gets sick, and they drop out. This way, you have a responsibility, and if you can't do it, then it's your responsibility to pull somebody else in who can take over that role. An awful lot of people, and I've done it myself, want to make a change and make a difference, so we give so much – and we have to really look at well-being and health from every perspective, including financial health. It is important not to drain yourself here – and equally making sure that the project itself is healthy.

You don't have to have be in menopause to be ready for this kind of thing, but I do think it is aimed at 45-plus, when women are ready to be collaborative, to be in a community and to work with co-operation. They're not feeling in competition, as maybe they did before, either with men or for jobs, but can really get in touch with their true self. That's the opportunity menopause gives us; the shift at that age – it's bringing together experience and wisdom, to become the Wise Woman. Because that's really where we're going; that's the next stage of our lives. The menopause should be welcomed and acknowledged as a rite of passage – a very healthy rite of passage – that we don't look at as the end but in fact the beginning.

I did a TEDx talk on the return of the Wise Woman in 2012, where I spoke about how it's time for us women crones to move into our power. I said in the talk that it's time for us to step up and create a world of co-operation – between women and men, science and spirituality, the old and the young, the environment and human beings, national politics and the true values of constituents. We Wise Women must guide the way to a template for the future where we can live together in peace and harmony, sustainability, growing our food and caring for our land. And teaching our young the power of good nutrition and the values that will bring them a happiness that isn't based on computer games or celebrity culture. We need a future where we can create communities that care for each other and where integrity, authenticity, courage, peace and love are the centre of our lives and the centre of our world.

One person I have had a huge amount of respect and time for is Dadi Janki, who was the head of the Brahma Kumaris. Sadly, she died earlier this year, at the age of 104, but even at an advanced age she continued travelling the world working for peace. She's been a great teacher of mine and an inspiration. Brahma Kumaris means 'Daughters of God' and they are the only women-led spiritual organisation in the world. This is because the man who founded Brahma Kumaris, eighty-odd years ago, said there will come a time for women's leadership – and of course the Dalai Lama said more recently that it is women of the West who will save the world. So, there are a lot of expectations for us women of a certain age – us Wise Women. Then there are the Thirteen Grandmothers – indigenous grandmothers who have come together from all over the world to share their wisdom and prayers. They meet regularly, although they are getting very old now, to look at the future. They dreamt each other in and they talk about, 'How do we create a world for the seven generations to come?' (Indigenous people generally talk about the seven generations to come.) I think we women of the West have to get back in touch with that side of ourselves. For me, postmenopause is the time to be the Wise Woman.

There weren't a lot of role models for my generation, really, and I lost a lot of my friends, my peers, who have died – like Anita Roddick, and Gabrielle Roth, who created the Five Rhythms, and others who passed away. I feel that those of us who have made it through and are still here, like myself, and who are healthy and have the energy, are here for a purpose and we shouldn't waste the privilege of still being alive and healthy and creative. We should use that energy for positive change.

As I said in my TEDx talk, I believe it's up to the women elders from all societies and backgrounds to show the way to a new paradigm based on spiritual values. It's vitally important for women to step up and take the lead in this transformation of society, where human beings are going to be equal brothers and sisters, walking shoulder to shoulder – whether it's in politics, in business, in community – and we women have to take the lead. We Wise Women have to show the way. We need to find a state of peace within us, where we stay calm and balanced, where we can project a sense of love and creativity to those we engage with. It's then up to us to live within our own co-operative world.

I think it's always important for women to mutually support each other, at any age – right from little girls in the playground. Even there you see it: she was my best friend, now she's not my best friend, and now she is again. We have to get over that as we get older, and that's about the Sky Dancer in my seven; it's about being graceful with relationships. It's very interesting for me now, being way past menopause, opening a café in a small town and meeting a lot of people that I wouldn't normally and seeing in all of them, in everybody I meet, something really special. We have women's gatherings here once a month, which are a cross-section of all different kinds of women – mostly 45 to 75, but not entirely. We've done a number of things about the menopause at those gatherings. The women here can't wait to connect and speak and share their stories. It's only the nonsense of societal norms that keeps people closed up.

Older women have a lot to give to society and should be listened to and taken much more seriously – as they indeed are in many indigenous tribes. It's the older women who are the leaders: spiritual leaders, shamans and community leaders. We need to do more of that here, and not just older women. Our small town of 5,500 now has a female mayor, and suddenly the women really are making decisions and doing things. It's fantastic. I'm not going to take credit for it – it's just perfect timing for me. I think the reason I'm in Wincanton is because I'm part of what's going on here, which is about living within a community where we can create shift and difference in many ways. Somerset has a tradition of so-called witches, who were mostly the wise women, many of whom were killed very brutally – including in Wincanton. So, 500 years ago in this place, we didn't have any power; and now we're back, and we do have power – but power in a way which is inclusive, for the men, for the children, for everybody. That's why I believe I'm here in this ancient space.

I think it's important to constantly see how we can transform ourselves and continue to grow, right up until we can't any more. Now in my early seventies, I'm still opening new businesses, I'm still creating new things,

I still have relationships, and I go to music festivals and I hang out with my grandchildren ... We don't stop at a certain age. I think age is just in the mind – and in the body to a degree, but then we say, 'OK, if this is a time of change, how can I live now in a better way and treat my body with more respect?' And that's what the menopause gives us: that sort of pause. It's just a pause, and then: I'm ready now to go forward. It's a very exciting time with a whole new future ahead of us.

Entrepreneur, PR legend, author and champion of women's empowerment – **Lynne Franks** has been a trailblazer her entire life. A successful self-made woman, Lynne left school at 16 and by the age of 21 had started Lynne Franks PR. This grew to become one of the most prestigious public relations firms in the UK and Lynne was the driving force behind London Fashion Week. She is the founder of SEED – Sustainable Enterprise and Empowerment Dynamics – which is based on her globally renowned *The SEED Handbook*, the first book to write about how women could start their own sustainable businesses based on feminine values. She initiated McDonald's UK and Europe's women's leadership network and has delivered programmes in partnership with The Prince's Trust, the World Bank and UNESCO. She is currently developing SEED programmes for women refugees and rural women in the Middle East, has opened the first SEED Hub in Somerset and is launching a new Women's Community site, www.seedhub.club.

20

The Menopause Café Story and Conversations

The Menopause Café, founded by **Rachel Weiss**, is a safe, open space for everyone to explore what menopause means to them, regardless of their gender or stage of life. Rachel shares her inspiration and vision for the movement, followed by a series of real Menopause Café conversations.

How to start a worldwide movement by watching TV: the Menopause Café story

'What shall we watch tonight?' my husband Andy asked on a dark February night three years ago. 'How about that menopause programme with Kirsty Wark?' I suggested. So we watched *Menopause and Me*, little realising that this would change our lives, leading us to establish a charity, organise a festival and speak on TV, and to coverage in newspapers including the *Daily Mail* and the *Guardian*. How strange that life can turn on such small things as choosing which TV programme to watch.

But that was all far ahead. Back on the sofa, watching Kirsty, two things struck me: first, that the menopause was likely to happen to me soon, since the average age for women in the UK is 51; and second, nobody seemed to talk about it. All I knew was that my periods would stop, and I might experience hot flushes. The programme opened my eyes to a range of other possible symptoms, psychological as well as physical. 'I wonder if anyone would be interested in a Menopause Café, like a Death Café, just with a different taboo topic?' I said idly to Andy.

From my day job as a counsellor and coach, I know that 'It's good to talk'. Being listened to non-judgementally, with genuineness and empathy, doesn't change the challenges we face, but it does empower us to examine our responses, to choose our mindset and to explore our options, instead of feeling like helpless victims of circumstances. Through being heard and accepted, we know that we are not alone, and we grow.

I had facilitated several Death Cafés in our hometown of Perth, Scotland. These are pop-up events, where people, often strangers, gather to drink tea, eat cake and talk about death. The Death Café movement was started by Jon Underwood and Sue Barsky-Reid in London in 2011, with the aim of 'increasing awareness of death with a view to helping people make the most of their (finite) lives'. It spread worldwide, tapping into people's need to learn through storytelling and connection. Could the same model work with this different taboo subject? Also, as an ex-Girl Guide, 'Be Prepared' is my motto: I don't cope well with the unknown; I like to be in control, to be informed before something happens, so I wanted to know more about the menopause before it happened to me – and I thought that maybe some other women would too, as might their partners and their colleagues.

I mooted the idea on Facebook and the response was overwhelming, including, crucially, from Gail Jack and Lorna Fotheringham, who offered to help organise it. I contacted Jon Underwood, who kindly gave his permission for us to adapt the Death Café model; I booked a venue for the evening; Andy created a web page advertising the event and Grainger PR organised a press release. That's how Gail, Lorna and Andy and I ended up sitting in Blend Coffee Lounge on a light June evening, feeling nervous and waiting to see whether anyone would turn up.

We had received plenty of media interest, featuring on STV news (Scotland's free-to-air TV channel) twice and in the local papers, but would that translate into bums on seats? To our relief, it did. Twenty-eight people, including two men, attended our Menopause Café. One woman had heard me on the six o'clock news that evening. Her husband had turned to her and said, 'You need to go there.' So she jumped in the car and arrived for the last fifteen minutes. We had clearly tapped into a hidden need for conversations about the menopause. As we sat and read the feedback sheets later that night, three comments stood out:

Now I know I'm not alone.

Now I know I'm not going mad.

When are you holding the next one?

The next one? We hadn't thought beyond whether anyone would turn up for this one! But we'd done it once, so we could do it again. We put a date in the diary for October, booked Blend and created a Facebook group.

Why now?

If we'd tried Menopause Café five years earlier, I think it would have flopped. There was something about 2017 that made the time finally ripe in the UK for public, informal discussion of the menopause, for gathering and sharing stories rather than keeping it behind closed doors as a topic of shame. I believe my mother's generation, starting work in the 1960s, had to strive to be accepted in the workplace, so they downplayed the differences between men and women. This meant not talking about menstruation, which makes talking about menopause difficult. They were so keen to be seen as equals that they didn't give any indication of any difference that could be interpreted as weakness and bias employers against hiring or promoting women – just as a few decades earlier the prospect of an employee becoming pregnant would commonly stop them being hired or even allowed to continue working.

But in the 2010s, we were moving on from equality towards valuing diversity. We felt secure enough to name our biological differences and still be respected in the workplace. The #MeToo phenomenon empowered women to speak up about sexual harassment and abuse. People were beginning to talk about their experiences of domestic abuse and mental health issues. Brené Brown's 2010 TED talk captured the spirit of a generation by encouraging us to see vulnerability as necessary and laudable, building intimacy as well as leadership. To walk into a room of strangers and discuss intimate matters takes some courage; I have admiration for all those who do this at a Menopause Café.

Older women were also becoming more visible, in a positive way, no longer disappearing into dowdy frocks once they passed 50. They were living longer, many enjoying decades of good health postmenopause and continuing to work. The increased pension age in the UK was another factor in women aged 50-plus becoming the fastest-growing demographic in the workforce. Businesses were beginning to take note, aided by the 2017 government report on the economic impact of menopause. Celebrities started speaking about their menopause on national TV: Lorraine Kelly, Carol Vorderman, Andrea McLean and now serious documentary journalist Kirsty Wark.

Period poverty rose to national awareness and talk of periods opens the door to talk of what happens when periods stop. Social media has been another factor. It enabled word to spread via Facebook, Twitter and Instagram, driving people to our website, alerting them to local Menopause Café events and creating online communities where stories and information and questions are shared. With hindsight, I can see that the time was right, although back in 2017 I had no idea why my idea of creating space for conversations about the menopause was proving so popular.

What is a Menopause Café?

The Menopause Café model is simple: gather people with a common interest together and let them talk and listen to each other. From the start, we set out certain principles as a guide. Following the Death Café model, we stated that a Menopause Café should be:

in an accessible, respectful and confidential space;
open to all, regardless of gender or age;
with an agenda created by the participants, no expectations or experts;
with no intention of leading people to any conclusion, product or course of action;
on a not-for-profit basis;
alongside refreshing food and drink.

These principles have proved helpful as the movement has grown. We want anyone to be able to host a Menopause Café. No knowledge about the menopause is required – I had none when I started! What is useful is having some people skills, especially in facilitation. I am told that I underestimate the skills required: finding a venue, publicising the event, welcoming people, keeping conversations on topic, moving people on to other tables, preventing anyone dominating the conversation.

We produced a *Guide to Hosting a Menopause Café* – a mixture of essential principles and structure with tips to help the event be useful and run smoothly. We ask hosts to welcome everyone at the start and outline the above principles, to invite everyone to sit round the café tables in small groups and to start by saying what their interest in menopause is, and to bring the event to a close with a thank you. Sometimes we invite participants to briefly say to the whole group what they have appreciated about the event.

Initially I had included the *Law of Two Feet*: if you are not learning from or contributing to a conversation, it's your responsibility to get up and find another conversation by moving to another table. However, I discovered that British reserve mitigates against this, and people felt too inhibited to follow their own interests and needs. I learned that anxiety and depression are common symptoms of menopause, as is lack of confidence. As a result of participant feedback, we introduced ringing a bell every twenty minutes or so to encourage people to move to another table instead.

One of the men who attended our first Menopause Café told me that he had deliberately stayed at the same table for the whole evening, so that women could choose whether to join a mixed-gender table or not. Since then we have encouraged other male participants to do the same, because some women prefer to discuss menopause at women-only tables, at least initially.

The most common themes which emerge at Menopause Cafés are:

Issues around sleep disturbance: insomnia, tiredness, fatigue, lack of concentration and subsequent impact on work/home life.

Mood swings, anxiety and rage.

HRT: a general sense of confusion about HRT (types, efficacy, mode of delivery), lack of GP awareness and reluctance to prescribe.

Impact on family life and relationships.

Coping strategies: importance of self-care, exercise, nutrition, being kind to ourselves.

Sex, low libido, vaginal dryness and issues with bladder (urine leakage, weak pelvic floor).

Conversations generally start with the physical and may then move on to the more philosophical and existential questions around gendered ageism and the meaning of life as an older woman.

Why and how the Menopause Café model works

The Menopause Café model has several distinctive aspects. The agenda of any Menopause Café gathering is group-directed, rather than speaker-led. The Café is empowering for participants, follows a therapeutic model rather than a medical model, and it is open to all.

The emergent agenda, which is generated by the participants instead of being planned by the host, is crucial. The Death Café model originally included structure and set questions, but Sue Barsky-Reid, who co-facilitated the first one with Jon Underwood, suggested moving to a more open format: 'Otherwise the conversation can become about what the facilitator is interested in.' Sue and I are both counsellors, which means we are comfortable trusting the process. The best Menopause Café hosts know how to hold the *process* without influencing the *content* of the conversations.

'Educate, empower, enable' is the motto of the global volunteer movement Soroptimist International, which works to empower women and girls, and it also applies to the Menopause Café. It's more empowering to have a conversation with peers than an appointment with a professional, or to attend a talk. Group conversations help us explore and clarify our own thinking, since 'in such environments, solidarity and even humour permeate the interpersonal atmosphere', as Assistant Professor of Sociology Jack Fong notes in *The Death Café Movement: Exploring the Horizons of Mortality*. People gather in small groups, with a single starter question – 'What brought you here?' and an optional 'harvesting' round where everyone is invited to end by saying, 'What are you taking away?' The Menopause Café model values our individual experience together with our commonality; I feel this often-quoted phrase is particularly appropriate: 'Always remember that you are unique, just like everyone else.'

While recognising the importance of accurate information provided by the medical profession, Menopause Cafés follow a therapeutic rather than

medical model, empowering participants to seek out information themselves and draw their own conclusions. Our events encourage the ancient
use of oral storytelling and sharing experiences to gain knowledge and
wisdom. Topics range from the physical, such as symptom relief, to the
philosophical and political: 'What does it mean to be an older woman in
society today?' to the existential: 'What is the purpose of my life now?'

Room for different views of menopause

Jack Fong refers to the 'trinity' of the market, media and medicine. These,
he says, 'may only serve to maximise people's fear, anxiety and despond-
ency ... due to the neglect of existential themes'. This trinity tells us to see
menopause as a problem to solve, an illness to cure. But Menopause Cafés
encourage individuals to frame their own narrative, with themselves as
hero instead of victim, choosing their own path through this time of transition. There is no one right path or choice. Menopause Cafés take us out
of our echo chambers and social bubbles, mixing us with strangers whose
different worldviews can challenge, enrich and enlarge our own. Hearing
views that we realise we disagree with helps us to clarify our own stance.

An alternative to the view of menopause as a problem is to see menopause as a mystery. The two views can co-exist in a single Menopause Café,
with participants first swapping practical tips on how to cope with vaginal
dryness and then discussing the new mindset which this third stage of life
is giving them. Like parenting, falling in love, ageing and bereavement, you
can read about the menopause, but you don't *know* until you have experienced it yourself. As Richard Rohr says about suffering in *Falling Upward: A
Spirituality for the Two Halves of Life*, 'it will be nothing like we might have
imagined beforehand'. Rarely is there a linear path through the menopause:
'Like skaters we move forward by actually moving from side to side,' Rohr
says about maturing, and the same is often true of menopause. We need
to be patient, to sit and listen, to ponder these things in our hearts, to talk,
to read and then the way forward emerges. This is counter-cultural to the
quick-fix of the developed world and has more in common with the Zen-like
mystery of spirituality and paradox. A Menopause Café can provide a space
for this gentler, more meandering approach.

I've been surprised at the resistance we've received about the model,
with comments such as:

You should have speakers.

Why can't we have women-only spaces?

What if nobody talks?

You don't know what they'll say.

Using a Menopause Café to promote a business, whether as a menopause coach, a complementary therapist or a nutritionist, violates the principle of Cafés being held 'with no intention of leading people to any conclusion, product or course of action'.

Being inclusive is crucial. It allows us each to learn from those who have gone before us, which is why we especially value the presence of post-menopausal women. Men often dominate mixed-gender groups, but at a Menopause Café they come from a humbler perspective, to listen and learn. This creates a different dynamic, which empowers women. It enables them, having practised talking menopause in the safe environment of the Café, to have those conversations with their men at home and at work.

Menopause Cafés are not support groups, since they are open to all regardless of age and gender. We have nothing against groups exclusively for menopausal women, or speaker events, but these are not Menopause Cafés. Our 'no experts, no expectations' approach seems radical to some. It may result in some false facts being shared, but we trust that, like Wikipedia, these will be corrected in the group and by reading. The open entry fits our remit to 'increase awareness of the impact of the menopause on those experiencing it, their friends, families and colleagues, so that they can make conscious choices about this third stage of life'.

For all of these reasons, we decided to protect the name and principles of Menopause Café® by trademarking the name.

A worldwide movement

Over 3,500 people have attended a Menopause Café, as of February 2020, with more than 400 pop-up events held in Scotland, England, Wales, Northern Ireland, the Republic of Ireland, Canada, the US, Denmark and Kenya. About 2 per cent of the participants identify as male, and that proportion is increasing. We are a registered charity, with Kirsty Wark as our patron. We've won the Prime Minister's Point of Light Award and the Association of Scottish Businesswomen's Award for Commitment to the Community. Lorna and Gail have moved on, but our committee has grown to include Helen Kemp, Heather Borderie and Moira MacLeod, together with Andy and me. We are proud of what we have achieved together, showing the power of teamwork and empathy, despite family and work commitments and menopausal brain fog!

In 2018, we held the world's first Menopause Festival, #FlushFest. Participants at Menopause Cafés told us they wanted reliable information from experts in the field. We can't provide this at a Menopause Café, so we came up with a festival to 'break the taboo and have some fun'. It includes talks from a medic, inspirational speakers, creative workshops, cabaret evenings and stand-up comedy – because laughter is the best medicine. #FlushFest now aims to be an annual event.

To raise funds for the festival, the intrepid committee have ended up doing things we would never have imagined, like participating in the Perth Santa Run (thanks, 'Couch to 5K'), modelling ethical, honest, body-positive underwear (thanks, Molke), speaking at conferences and agreeing to write this chapter (thanks, Caroline, for encouragement and editing). Our voluntary work for Menopause Café has expanded and enriched our lives.

'Menopause Café at Work' is another unexpected offshoot. In January 2018, Scottish and Southern Energy (SSE) hosted a Menopause Café onsite at lunchtime. Over thirty employees turned up to discuss menopause with their colleagues. Many other organisations followed suit, including universities, health trusts and charities. A Menopause Café at Work serves as a springboard for action. It acts as market research, starting from the grassroots to discover what employees need, rather than a top-down decision. It often leads to menopause education for managers, menopause policies, speaker events and support groups. As we remind all our hosts, the impact extends beyond actual 'bums on seats' – seeing a Menopause Café advertised at work or in public is a catalyst for conversations with friends, family and colleagues, helping to reduce the stigma and increase awareness of the menopause.

The setting for a Menopause Café is important to create an inclusive yet boundaried space for conversation. We need to be contained enough to feel safe, yet not constrained. Professor Ray Oldenburg's notion of a 'third place' describes what we aim to create at a Menopause Café. Oldenburg defines third places as environments, such as pubs and hairdressers, which promote casual conversation between strangers. They are democratic spaces, free from the power of the expert or the status quo, be it government, celebrities or big pharma. Seventeenth-century London coffee houses were third spaces where citizens met to discuss and create their own ideas; they were seen as beds of dissent. However, I wonder whether our cafés are biased towards the chattering middle classes – and whether we are unwittingly choosing venues which perpetuate this. At the Menopause Café at the Scottish Trade Union Conference (STUC) in Perth in 2019 we heard from train drivers and others whose work environment makes it harder to change clothes or have immediate toilet breaks for flooding. Menopause Cafés at Work help to broaden our reach and inclusivity.

Some Menopause Café groups have evolved away from our model to become support groups, or to hold speaker events, or women-only groups. We are pleased to have provided a springboard for these groups to discover the needs of their community and to change to meet them.

Our aims for the immediate future are to include greater diversity of participants by gender, age, culture and class, to experiment with virtual Cafés in real time and to spread to more countries. In the longer term, our plan is to become redundant. I picture a time when the menopause is as ordinary a topic of conversation as pregnancy, puberty and other times when our bodies and hormones change. A time when there is no stigma attached to going through the menopause and support is provided at home and at work. And a world where women already know about common symptoms and what they can do to reduce them, instead of learning about menopause for the first time from a TV programme they happen to watch at the age of 50.

Menopause Café conversations

These conversations took place at the Menopause Café meeting in Perth at the end of January 2020.

Conversation 1: Sandra and Caroline

Sandra: I'm here because I am 53 and going through the menopause, and I'm looking for information. We're all just figuring it out as we go along, aren't we?

Caroline: Definitely. I was 46 when I first started skipping periods. I reached menopause at about 51 and am now dealing with postmenopause. What made you realise you might be in perimenopause?

Sandra: I was in my mid-forties and having very heavy periods, to the point where if I was making arrangements to go out for a day, or for a walk, I'd be saying, 'Oh I might not go today.' It did begin to limit me, which was annoying. I also suffer from very tight muscles in my back and I have begun to wonder if that is less to do with a sore back and more to do with the changes in hormones. I had anxiety for a long time as well, but that seems to have eased. I do a lot of meditation now, which I've found helps. For about the last year I'd say I am in the menopause. Though I'm a bit confused about when or what that is.

Caroline: My understanding is that menopause, in the medical definition, is when periods stop completely. So you are considered as having gone through menopause if you've not had a period for a year. But for me, and I think this is something that happens for other people too, menopause coincided with a stressful time personally, especially with my parents.

Sandra: So, you don't know then if some symptoms were to do with menopause or with that?

Caroline: Exactly. I was quite lucky with menopause symptoms. I didn't get heavy bleeding or anything, but lots of hot flushes, and what I noticed as well was the effect on sex.

Sandra: I don't suffer from dryness, but I have next to no desire, other than every now and then. My poor husband is very patient. We do discuss it now, but it's really hard when you don't have the information to do anything about it. I hadn't had hot flushes – one spell of them, which completely went away – but then all of a sudden in the past month or so I'm getting them regularly, to the point where I can feel my heart beginning to beat fast. I'll be perspiring and then suddenly that subsides and I start shivering.

Caroline: People don't really talk about that. They talk about getting really hot, but not the sudden cold. It's like when you've been out for a run – like this huge shot of energy has gone through and then it leaves you depleted. Are you still having the heavy periods?

Sandra: No. They got very light, and then a year ago I thought, 'Oh, that's it,' and then I had one very light one. Then there's been nothing since. I've lost track a bit, but I think that's pretty much a year now without. Maybe I can officially say I am in the menopause! My big question is, though, is this for evermore? You don't talk about the end of the menopause.

Caroline: My understanding is that some things continue. Some people find hot flushes continue, that they're just more sensitive in that way. Some people say they get through it and then that's it. And they notice greater clarity, for example, because of not having the hormonal changes.

Sandra: That would be good, because I did suffer from ups and downs. Even in the last week, I had two days' worth of feeling exceptionally happy, for no reason whatsoever. Nothing had changed, but everything seemed lovely, and then the next day I could feel myself beginning to go down. I don't suffer from depression normally, but I could feel my mood subsiding.

Caroline: Were there any other symptoms linked to that?

Sandra: Well, lots of hot flushes throughout the day, though I would say, today and yesterday, they are less intense. So I think there has been a hormonal thing going on there.

Caroline: There's so much we don't know about how our bodies work. When you're having periods, you take it for granted: 'Oh, it's that monthly thing.' But we understand so little about the subtleties and nuances.

Sandra: And all that 'Is this a symptom of hormones, or is this a symptom of life?' We just don't know.

Caroline: That's it. I feel that during my menopausal time I just kept on going: I didn't *feel* particularly stressed, but I think I was.

Sandra: Yes, I was similar. We'd just come back to this area after being away for twelve years. We'd moved to a new house, but we'd made a mistake with the one that we'd bought. And then my dad died suddenly, in a foreign country.

Caroline: Oh no ...

Sandra: Actually, that was a turning point for me, because I wanted so much to go to his funeral, because I had not been to see him for a long time, although we'd kept in touch. I ended up going there, and it was a stressor, but at the same time you get over it: I am a woman in her fifties and I can do these things now. People talk about almost a coming of age, it feels like that to me.

Caroline: With things I have been through with my relationship, and with both of my parents' deaths, I feel like I can probably deal with pretty much anything that's thrown at me now. There are obviously things that are unimaginable, but I have a sense of that coming of age, definitely.

Sandra: Out of all the negative things that are happening with menopause, that is a positive, isn't it: that sense of yes, we can deal with things now, and enjoying the fact that we are this age. Maybe it's not a negative thing, it is a positive thing.

Conversation 2: Helen and Caroline

Helen: I had a TAH/BSO [a total abdominal hysterectomy and removal of both ovaries and fallopian tubes] aged 41, due to endometriosis, heavy, painful periods, fibroids and ovarian cysts. As having children had never been on my radar screen, I was more than happy to have the surgery and I thought after the obvious post-op recuperation period, I'd be back firing on all cylinders again.

However, I had post-operative complications. I didn't heal properly internally, and every two to three months I would bleed, and then be referred back to the hospital. I was concerned at the time that it was recurrence of the endometriosis. A year after surgery, and six months after returning back to work, I had a breakdown and resigned from my job.

In the weeks after the hysterectomy, my depression returned with a vengeance. I'd navigated depression since my mid-teens, and assumed it was just another blip. However, it didn't pass, and I started to become anxious, have panic attacks, suicidal ideation, and an eating disorder that I had conquered back at university also returned. My joints became sore and stiff, I had gingivitis twice (for the first time in my life), I was getting by on two to three hours' sleep a night, experienced mood swings, brain fog, daily bouts of nausea, and my hair continued to fall out. And, of course, I was still having episodes of bleeding, which were eventually identified as being a result of GSM [genitourinary syndrome of menopause]. But back then, I was just going around in endless circles, becoming more desperate.

Caroline: Why were the doctors not saying these could be symptoms relating to the hysterectomy?

Helen: I have no idea, because I saw the same surgeon. I mean, he was a fantastic surgeon, but no one seemed to join any of the dots. It reached a point where he said, 'Well, I can't do another chemical cauterisation, you need to have more surgery,' and I said, 'No, I'm not having more surgery.' I don't know why it was missed, every time I would be examined ... And that was when I went on HRT.

Caroline: So how did you know to ask for HRT?

Helen: It was my husband. Immediately after I'd had surgery, he said, 'Aren't you going on HRT?' But because my mother had had the same surgery at the same age, and she hadn't taken HRT and said she didn't need it, I think there was something in the back of my mind: 'Well, why would I need HRT?' I didn't link all the symptoms together. I think it takes someone from the outside looking in. Also, I think there's a stigma with the mental health side of it. Because I'm very stubborn, I'm very persistent, I just thought it was a matter of 'I just need a bit more sleep, I'm just tired, I'm working too hard ...'

Caroline: It's easy to think that it's us, that it's an individual thing, of 'If only I could cope better with this, or do that.'

Helen: Certainly talking about it has helped – that's why I attended the first Café, to try and see how others were coping and what worked for them. I think actually being part of the Menopause Café – I joined the steering group after that inaugural Café – has been pivotal in, if you like, my whole recovery journey, because it gave me a purpose then. And I think if you've got an interest that you are invested in you just naturally go towards it and it's almost like finding your tribe. There's a sense of togetherness, a collective kindness almost, as well as compassion, because we're all more or less there or have been there.

Caroline: An understanding, fellow feeling ...

Helen: I think it's validating, because some of the symptoms can appear so vague and so completely unrelated. I was talking to a lady and she said, 'Gosh itchy skin,' and she didn't realise it was one of the, I think, thirty-four symptoms of menopause.

Caroline: One thing I have been thinking about is that when I was in my late twenties, I had chronic panic attacks, which I gradually dealt with, but actually it's interesting that they *didn't* come back with menopause for me.

Helen: I started, and other people as well, to have panic attacks at the beginning of menopause. And I wonder if that's the body's reaction to the hormone fluctuations. Some women seem to get very bad migraines at the start.

Caroline: I had really bad migraines during pregnancy, and they came back again around perimenopause.

Helen: Yes, a sort of a hormone sensitivity. My feeling is that some women have a real sensitivity, like with PMDD [premenstrual dysphoric disorder], for example. Also suicidal ideation – the number of women who experience that but who don't want to talk about it. For example, I wouldn't walk over bridges for a while. I used to sit through meetings and the whole time I was thinking, 'I want to die.' And this is only three years ago. You think, well, where does that come from? I think it's very confusing, but then you start to talk to other women and they say, 'Yes, I couldn't go driving, because I wanted to drive my car off the road ...' But talking helps. The Menopause Café movement is game-changing.

Conversation 3: Mary, Anna, Maggie and Caroline

Mary: So why am I here? I'm now 66 and well through the menopause. I'm just here to prove there is life after. You do come out the other side – with a few hiccups, but you do come out the other side.

Anna: I've been before and it was mostly actually to ask Rachel about having a stall at #FlushFest, because I'm part of a local running group. I feel that there's not enough emphasis on older people, especially women, doing any kind of activities. My perception was that we're encouraged to be very gentle on ourselves. But we can still do the same things, despite menopause and its problems.

Caroline: And I think, actually, exercise can be of help during menopause.

Anna: That's my personal experience. I realise that exercise isn't for everybody. Not everybody can exercise because they may have other physical problems. And it's not the cure-all, but I think to some degree, there are things that it can help with.

Mary: I'd go with that. I don't run, except very, very occasionally for the bus, but I do a lot of walking. I find if I'm not feeling right, then I take myself out for a walk. It's just being outside. I can't walk away from the problems, because I carry them with me, but walking somehow keeps it under control. I've always walked, including during menopause, and the more my mind gets upset, the more I want to walk. Also postmenopause, you're more likely to get osteoporosis: get out there and walk, you're getting your bones working.

Maggie: Well, I am in the thick of the menopause being 53. I'm sweating, I've got restless legs at night. But again, I go walking to try and combat feeling stuck indoors, because I'm single. I walk the dog miles. When I say at the doctor, 'How long does this last for?' he says, 'How long is a piece of string?'

Mary: Yes, everybody's different.

Anna: For me, sometimes symptoms have felt overwhelming at the time and it does feel better when I go for a run. When you see what women have written on online forums, it seems that if they're in the thick of it, whatever symptoms are worst will just overwhelm them completely, and they feel really lost. It seems like the forums are a sort of scream room for some women. It's sad that's the case.

Maggie: With the hot flushes it's also embarrassing. I could be in the middle of church or in the middle of a shop or in the middle of somebody's house and it starts. I feel like my face just goes 'whoof' and I think, 'Oh no.' It's like someone is pushing the gas button and the ignition has been lit and the sweating begins. And I've said to friends, 'Is your heating on?' and they've said, 'No, it's not.' And I say, 'Well mine is, and it doesn't have an off button.'

Caroline: So, is that the most worrying symptom for you?

Maggie: No. I can put up with sweating because you can always open a window, or take off a jumper. The biggest problem for me is restless leg syndrome. It starts when I go to bed. I usually lie on my right side, then my hip starts aching and then my legs start aching. Both of my legs are aching the whole night. I toss and turn and toss and turn all night. And I wake like I've not had any sleep and I'm exhausted all day.

Mary: Have you been able to get any help for that?

Maggie: It's just trial and error. The doctor tries me on this pill and that pill, and it works for a while and then it loses its effectiveness, because you get used to them. It's called augmentation.

Mary: For me, it was more the mental thing. I just felt very confused. Making decisions was more difficult than usual. I couldn't take things in. My husband got very frustrated because he would tell me something and I just wouldn't be able to retain it. He found that very hard to understand: 'Do I have to tell you over and over again?' 'Yes, you do at the moment.' Then the problem was when I came out and was able to retain information, he couldn't get out of that habit. I had to remind him that I was no longer menopausal.

Anna: I'm glad you said that, because when I first started off, about a year and a half ago, I had just started a new job. It's not a particularly skilled job, but there was a worksheet that I would have to tick stuff off, and I'd forget to tick it off or I'd look at it and I just couldn't make sense of what I was reading. I got to the point that they were reading it out to me and it depressed me so much, because I'm wanting to say, 'I'm not stupid!' And then they continued the habit and sometimes they still do it. They're the nicest guys you could work for, but they don't realise they're doing it. You know?

Maggie: When you were in the middle of it, Mary, did you ever think it was never going to go away?

Mary: Yes, I thought I was losing my mind. I really began to wonder if I was getting early onset Alzheimer's or something.

Anna: That's how I found it. Initially I started going on a lot of forums. You go on and you ask a question and somebody else is, 'Yeah, I've had that,' and you think, 'Oh thank God for that'.

Mary: Because you do feel it's just you.

Anna: You just feel so alone. And there's this fear, there's anxiety. And you can't explain it. But at the same time, all these women are in the same position. I don't know how our mothers coped. My mother went to her bed for about a year. And now I understand why.

Caroline: I think that's the thing, isn't it: maybe they weren't coping, but because it wasn't talked about, people thought, perhaps, that women were coping when actually it was really difficult.

Maggie: Even when I was young, I remember my stepdad saying, 'Don't upset your mother, it's a bad week.' And I didn't know what the 'bad week' was until I started getting the 'bad week' and I was like, 'Oh'. Because of PMT my mum would be crying in front of my stepdad and I'd be in tears for no reason. And my stepdad would say, 'What's the matter with you?' He'd say, 'Oh, bloody women, I'm off out to the pub.' And off he'd go, out the door he'd go.

Mary: I remember my mum sitting there, and she took to wearing cardigans, and when she was sitting at the table all of a sudden the cardigan would come off. Then five minutes later the cardigan went back on, and twenty minutes later it came back off again. I think with menopause it was: it happens to everybody, it's part of life. Get on with it. One of the things that really bugged me most about the menopause when I was going through it, was that people would say about the sweats, the risk of osteoporosis, the mental stuff and all the rest of it. But the one thing that was never touched on was the fact that it affects your pelvic floor muscles. I've had slight urinary incontinence but that was never mentioned and it really annoyed me.

Caroline: It is interesting that within a taboo subject of menopause, there are some things that are more taboo than others. Some things that it's OK to kind of 'own' and own up to and others not.

Mary: And incontinence is not. Everybody is different, but I remember reading an interview with somebody and they mentioned it and I thought, 'Thank God, it's not just me.' As Anna said: it's not just me. And that is something you don't get until you are in a group where you can talk. It's not something you tend to talk about in front of men, but fair enough, for them it's hard too. I sometimes think the men need to get together and talk. But get a man to talk ...! Not when he's my generation anyway. But this does help. When I first started coming, it was partly about libido and sex and I wanted to find if I was the only one experiencing that, or if it was a general thing – and it was about 50:50. But then as I went through menopause and came out the other side – and I couldn't tell you exactly when I realised I'd come out the other side – but as I get older I keep just coming along to say: I'm here to prove there's life afterwards. And I find it ironic that actually I am now feeling better than I have in years.

Rachel Weiss is a counsellor and a coach at Rowan Consultancy in Perth, Scotland, which helps people live more satisfying lives. Rowan Consultancy offers counselling and coaching alongside workplace mediation and training. She is also the founder of the Menopause Café charity, a social franchise supporting pop-up events worldwide. Since turning 50, she has taken up learning Spanish and reluctantly running. She enjoys walking, knitting, tweeting and sleeping. To learn more about Menopause Café see www.menopausecafe.net or follow on Facebook www.facebook.com/menocafe17 or Twitter or Instagram @Menopause_Cafe. Find Rachel on Twitter at @Rowan_Rachel.

21

Loving Life Now

Olympic gold-medal-winning athlete, first Black woman to win gold for Great Britain, first woman Vice Chair of Sport England and Patron of Adoption UK, **Tessa Sanderson CBE** explores how her attitudes to health, exercise and family helped her through the menopause.

I was probably 49 when I started to notice the symptoms. I was going out and doing a lot more talks and public appearances and regularly being around big crowds. I found I was perspiring a lot, and after eating I was feeling bloated. Of course, if a room is crowded, you think, 'It's a bit warm in here' – when it wasn't that warm. I was also coming out in rashes between my fingers, like little bubbles or water pimples. They'd itch like hell. But to be honest, I ignored it, because I just thought: 'Oh, it's one of those things, you're a bit nervous – it's a nervous rash.' Then one time it carried on for a couple of days and I went to my GP and said: 'I've got this flaming rash on my fingers, it's making my fingers swell up, so what is it?' and he said to me: 'It's all down to the menopause.'

I thought, well, men always say that, or doctors will link it with that because I'm coming up to my fifties. I suppose the shock of it was that to me, menopause was something you had in your sixties. I thought, 'How can that be? I'm not old enough yet.' It's maddening, because once you talk about menopause, people think you're old. Some friends would say, 'Ah Tessa, you're there, at the menopause.' If you're feeling a little sick, it's: 'Oh, it's the menopause, girl!'

When they said about getting old, it made me think. I remember analysing: 'I feel fine in myself. OK, I'm getting hot, maybe a little bothered, and when I'm talking to someone, not short-tempered, but ...' Maybe it was right, it was all linked to menopause. I wondered, was that one of the reasons why I couldn't conceive? I had all this sort of stuff in my mind, but I never thought for a minute, 'Oh you're too old, you're getting to that age, you've got to sit back now and that's it.'

I think women have this fear factor. They are frightened of approaching *that* age. They think: 'I'm going to feel so different, my life's going to change. That's it, my life's finished.' I don't agree with that, because I don't think it's true. Women in their sixties now are stronger, dealing with a lot of stuff, and happy in what we're doing. And I think we should all try and adopt this attitude. There is so much more to go for. Don't be embarrassed about it, either. Men and boyfriends nowadays, they watch pregnancies, they watch you giving birth to your babies, so don't clam up about menopause. When I went to my functions, I always carried a fan and a little face cloth, so I could sneak in the loo and dampen my neck, put it under my arm. When I got home at night, I'd have a tepid shower, to cool the whole body down. And then it's all fine. If you make a bigger thing of it than it is, then that can make it more difficult.

When you wake up in the morning, sometimes you might feel like rubbish, but if you look in the mirror, you have your shower, then you feel much more refreshed, and I'm like, let's go put a bit of slap on. I never go outside without lipstick on, never – unless I'm rushing for the school run. You probably don't feel 100 per cent alive, but you look OK. And you've got to feel inside as well as outside that you're OK. I think it's a true saying: smile and the world smiles with you. Even if you're aching inside, if you're smiling, that other person doesn't really know what's going on, and that smile has boosted everything up.

One of the things to do is exercise. I'm 63 now and I feel it's important not stop my life from being active. Walking is a massive must, because there are so many different forms of walking you can do. Power walking is fantastic, or just walk at your own pace – get a little group to meet up and walk around a big park twice. It's great, because that helps loosen up the mind, loosen up the body. I've done aerobics too, and now I'm doing a lot of body combo with this fantastic teacher that I work with. I try to keep my body toned.

A lot of stretching and exercises for stomach are good, because if you keep your stomach in shape, that takes away a lot of the bloating. Some people hate sit-ups, but it's exercise you can do in your house. Even if you're doing five or six sit-ups, twice or three times a week, that's great. Similarly with jogging: not everybody likes to jog, but first you go into a walking routine and then you start the jog, so you build up to it. Just get active and that way I think your whole body, your whole persona, starts to feel fitter. You feel healthier, your mind's starting to work on a different level. I mean, I don't feel like I did when I was competing, but I feel I could still throw a javelin. Not as far, but I still go and run around a track, and I swim now. I'm not saying to go out and be overly active, but exercise is a key factor, I feel, for menopause.

You really have to look at your diet, too. From my track-and-field days to now, I've changed that so much. It's about recognising your body and thinking: 'I don't have to be so strong and powerful any more, all I need is just to make sure I keep supple, I keep healthy.' I want to be at this frame. I don't have to train seven days a week, or anything like that, so I did change my diet. I eat a lot more fish. I didn't cut out red meat – I eat steak and things like that as well – but my first choice is very much fish, and I've learned that oily fish is good. In my competition days it used to be a lot of Caribbean cooking: rice and peas, chicken, curried goat – a lot of this heavy food. But my build needed to be powerful and strong, and that made me feel like I had enough energy, enough stamina, to do what I was doing.

I didn't think about HRT. But I didn't have any of the aches and pains that some people do. Some people feel that they can cope better with it, but for me, I thought, 'I really don't need that.' I think one of the things you've got to do is to understand your body and know what sort of treatment you would probably like – which doesn't have to mean medicinal treatment. It may reach a point of talking to your doctor about HRT, but up until then I think there are a lot of things you can do.

I never heard my mum talk about or even mention the word menopause when I was growing up. Never. In those days it was a real taboo. Nobody talked about stuff like that because it was deemed as, 'You can't go there.' You'd have to pluck up a lot of courage to talk about it. With my sister we talked about period pains, and all that, but this word we didn't even know of.

I had a very lively and a very caring family background. My mum was a hairdresser; my dad was a sheet-metal worker. They were very normal but made sure that the right things were in place for you to learn and understand. They tried to make sure that we didn't miss out on anything, although they didn't have any bucks, any money. For example, every Friday, we'd call that fish and chips night and my dad would make sure we had pie and chips or fish and chips and a Mars bar when he came home from the pub. Even if we went broke, he'd make sure that all four of us (I've got two brothers and one sister) were settled and feeling like the rest of the world. With my athletics, when my family first heard about it, they thought: 'This is crazy, this is just a fad.' It was the 1960s, and racism was going on right, left and centre. You've got to get into nursing, they thought, because nursing was the thing for Black people then. I went to see a hospital, and I thought, 'Forget that. Too much blood for me here.' It was a great career to do, but I knew it wasn't for me. But afterwards, when my teacher came and talked to my mum about athletics, they thought it was heavenly, so they supported me. My background was very solid in that. I knew that I had the support of my family. But also they were very realistic, and my confidence came too from having been told by my family that there comes a time when you have to move into areas where you probably feel you're not good enough to do them, but you are, and unless you have a go, you're not going to know. I was always one who wanted to know things, do things, go into areas where people never went. In those days, I remember saying to my brothers, 'When you grow up, don't just go to Jamaica, go somewhere else, try and see the world.' I wanted to do that.

I went back to Jamaica in 1974 for the first time, when I would have been 18 or 19, to see my grandmother who I grew up with. It was fascinating, because I wanted to see the world. And I do think that having that background of travel, my athletics, the support, being competitive – and it doesn't have to be sport, it can be being competitive in your life, in your job – has made me like this. I would teach my children to be competitive, because I do feel life is competitive. That's taught me not to be fearful. It's taught me that if it doesn't happen the first time – like when I had IVF – you try again. When it didn't happen the second time, I cried, but I got over it. Because you accept that it's life.

I think it all comes from family background and knowing that you have confidence in your family, and your family has confidence in you. That and setting challenges for yourself. It's important you set them yourself, and that you want to do these things – that nobody's setting them for you, or you're doing it because it's a fad, because then you don't enjoy it as much. And some of them can be tough, because life is not easy.

We see now there is still a lot of racism going on, and that's sad. In my competition days, a lot of the times I didn't have blatant racism, but I experienced blatant bias. I think, when you're Black, sometimes you have to be stronger. But things have changed, because there are a lot of mixed-race people now, and people are more amenable and sensible. I don't think you have to fight, fight, fight the battle any more. But I do think that being there in those early days, it helped your mind be a little bit stronger, and I'm sure it prepared me. As Black women, we've had to fight our way through, especially if you were in an environment where it was predominantly white.

My mum, my sister and I behave like three sisters. My sister and I never have a big quarrel and she's now 66. In all the life we've gone through we've just talked about any and everything. When the doctor told me that the IVF had failed, I remember stopping my car by the bus stop and I just started crying. I rang her up and I said, 'I've just had my second IVF and the doctor's rung with the result, and my eggs didn't fertilise.' I was so tearful, and she was saying, 'Come home, come home.' I rang my mum in Jamaica and told her about it. She is very Gospel, very godly, she's like a guardian angel. She just said to me: 'That's God's way, my child, you know.' But yes, I felt really heartbroken. I found myself saying to my mother and sister, 'How can that be? I don't do drugs, I eat healthily, you guys have had all your family ... what is it?' Then I started looking at athletics and thinking, 'Did I go on too long? Did I push my body too much?' And then I remembered that when I'd injured my back, in 1990, I'd had to have a steroid injection because I'd blown my disc. Everything was coming into my mind – all the awful things that one could think of, everything that was negative. I thought, 'Why? To me, I feel good, I feel perfect, so why isn't this happening?'

Then after long chats with my family, especially my mum and my sister, and my then partner, I thought, 'Two rounds of IVF is enough. What can they do? This body of mine, it just doesn't want to do that.' So I just thought, 'I've had enough of that, I'm not going to upset myself any more. Let's move on.' My mum and sister pointed out that there are other processes, like adoption. At first I thought, no: it was an option, but not for me, because you want this – you want to be a mum, you want to have children. But then I sat down and thought about it and realised, 'Well that's just as good.' So I looked at all the options. I was way past 40 then, and I so wanted children.

It all came together when I met my husband, Dens. We've been married for nine years. I remember the first date that we had. We went out to have something to eat, and we were talking about all this stuff, like has he got any children, and he said, well, yeah, he's got two boys, but he was never married. And he said to me, 'You haven't, have you?' and I said, 'No.' And I just found myself telling him everything. I said, 'Dens, this is what I'd really like. I'd love to adopt because I really want children. My whole family, they've had kids. My sister's had kids, my brother's had children, and I really like children. What do you think?' And he said: 'I'll support you whatever you want to do.' And I thought, 'You know what, this person is my ideal person.'

I'd known Densign since 1984, at the Olympics. We both lived in Wolverhampton at an early age, but we never saw each other then. We'd see each other now and then through competition, but in 1984, we really sort of met and were close – never dated or anything, but I fancied him like crazy! After I won my medal, he was coming out of the canteen and I was going in, and as he passed me he said, 'Did you win, then?' And I went, 'Yeah,' and he went, 'Yeah, right!' and he carried on and walked off! Later, when I was in the physio room, he'd heard by then, and he was like, 'Oh Tessa, I'm so sorry ...' In a way I don't really blame him, because everybody thought Fatima [Whitbread] was going to win, or Tiina Lillak, and I was ranked fourth going out there.

After the 1984 games, he went back to where he was and I was in London, and we dated different people. Then for my fiftieth birthday, because we'd been talking, I rang him up and I said, 'Dens, I'm having my fiftieth birthday, would you like to come?' And he said he'd love to come but he couldn't. So I thought OK, it's not a problem. By this time I was really being coiffured and making sure that things are looking happy. Never mind menopause, I was looking at a peak.

We didn't speak again for a little while, and then I was in Jamaica and he sent me a message on New Year's Eve, wishing us Happy Christmas, Happy New Year. I was there with my mum and I remember I showed her and she said, 'Oh, isn't that lovely.' Then for my fifty-first birthday – because we'd been talking and he'd been coming to London – I picked up the phone and said, 'Look, my birthday's coming up again, would you like to ...' I didn't even finish the word and he said: 'Oh yeah, love to come.' That was it, and we've been dating ever since.

I was 56 when we got the twins. The whole process started round about 53. Dens and I, we wanted to get married first. The adoption process wasn't easy, but it wasn't overly hard. I'm glad that we went through it, because we had six weeks' training, counselling, seeing what adoption involves. I think it's really important that one gets to know the agencies and that you go to talk with people who have fostered or adopted. That way, it made things easier. I explained to Dens what he would have to do as well. One of things is making sure that your family is involved. My sister came with me to the meetings, but sometimes that could be tough, because she would have to rush off to work. But she did it, and that's important – to have someone close like that. I went through that process willingly and I felt it was the right thing to do. Both Dens and I felt it was the right thing to do.

I did change adoption agencies, because we were nearly there with one child, but things didn't work out with what the agency was asking of us. I remember I came out of the meeting in tears, but it didn't stop me, it didn't deter me. So I moved on and joined another agency, who were absolutely marvellous. I couldn't wish for better. They nurtured, they explained everything. They made sure you realised that you'd have to change your home a little bit – because we were having young babies – and were you willing to do that ... They'd call on you ad hoc to check; it didn't matter what time. Sometimes they'd tell you when they were coming, other times they were just there.

When we did get the children, it was a matter of remembering the mind of a child again. The twins were three months old, a boy and a girl. You had to nurture them, you had to make sure they were fed on time. Getting up in the early hours wasn't really a major task because Dens and I travelled a lot, so we know what it's like to get up at two o'clock, three o'clock in the morning. It was really exciting times. We'd prepared this room, bought two fantastic Edwardian cots for them, and Dens was busy doing the filming and all that sort of thing ... From then till now it's been our world; it's the best thing that could have happened.

A couple of people did say to me at the time, 'Are you mad?' Because you're over 50 and it's hard work. I found the energy because I put my mind to it. I kept myself fit and so did my husband. We were very active in what we were doing. We really wanted this to happen. You've got to want it to happen – it's not something where you can change your mind in a couple of months because it's hard work. But if your mind's set on doing it, you're happy doing it. We love changing the nappies! It was great getting up and giving the twins a feed, and when they walked, and being in the little bouncy cot ... Every little challenge. It was a showing-off stage, I suppose. The nightmare was having a twin pushchair. Oh please. I think that was the worst bit: getting in and out of shops. Especially if I went out on my own. You're standing there waiting for people to open the door, or you're trying to do it yourself. But I'm glad that we went through the tasks we had to before adopting, because we learned a lot about children, their behaviour. It teaches you how to behave, and also confidence. It's not about being temperamental: you have to make sure that you're calm even when you don't want to be.

The twins are 7 now. My little girl, she's very much a diva. My little boy, he's the gentleman. Ah, he's so clever. He will talk you through the earth, about planets, about Tyrannosaurus. Every day he's challenging me with new things in Maths, and I'm thinking, 'I don't know the hell about Maths, I hate it!' My little girl is catching up, too. She never wants his help, of course. She loves music, she speaks great. It's all good. But they fight like hell! Something like having young children does make you think about menopause. Because you've got to keep active, you've got to set yourself challenges. If you don't, you'll just be living in a bottle. And that's not the way to live at all.

What I have learned from my experience of menopause is that this is one of the things that women will have. Whatever happens, women will have it. Be it small, large ... It's something we must learn not to be embarrassed about. If you talk about it more, it feels better. It's like having a really bad headache – you don't sit and suffer. Talk about it – talk with close friends, have a laugh about it. When my friend joked that I brought my fan everywhere, we'd laugh about it. Why not? It's part of life.

One of the most important points that I want to make is that I love life now. I loved life before, but I feel great now, I really do. I feel that my body isn't overworked, it's not harassed. My skin is better now than in my young days. And I think that is about nurturing. I'm not into this big cleanse, moisturise, all this scrubbing. I exfoliate now and then, but that's it. I've never had botox. And I feel better now than I've ever felt, thank God. I think I'm a much more balanced person, with my whole body, and I'm not frightened of the next age, which is going to be 64. Yeah, of course, sometimes I think, 'God, I'll be 64, it's 35 years since I won the javelin, what am I doing?' But the thing is, I'm just taking every day as it comes. If I feel tired in the morning, I tell myself, 'OK, I'm tired, but I've got to do this school run.' I know people think it's utter madness. But I do find time to relax and time to set challenges. I find time to be in that nice, friendly, relaxed zone. Don't let people bog you down with depression – it's too tough out there. Just be in that happy mood; you can't be all the time, but when you can be.

I suppose I have my family around, I have a wonderful husband, and I have two fab kids. Every day there are new challenges. Some of them, if I can't do them, then sod it! Let's do something that I can really do. I'm a mother first and foremost, and I love being a mum. Even the cooking I get to like now and then. I like to experiment with different things, not just Caribbean meals, and if it doesn't work, I try again. But all of those are nice challenges. And I think that keeps my mind really healthy, happy. When I do feel a bit down, I accept it as I'm feeling a bit off that day. And if you do feel like you want to cry sometimes then, hell, you should. Then you can think, 'OK, I've done that now. I'm not going to cry because I feel like that any more. I've done my crying; I'm going to get on with this.' And if the menopause is hurting, then cry a little bit, but then you get the paper and flick it over and think, 'OK, let me read up about this thing: why is it making me feel like this?'

Yes, I am enjoying life very much. I'm doing all these different things, like hosting events. There's been so much more since 1984. I have done so many things it's untrue. I did the swimming for Stand Up To Cancer – I mean, I drank sea water for Britain, but it was a wonderful cause. I'm very much into working my fitness routine. I'm still doing TV. Life is pretty active and I'm really liking it.

On 6 August 1984, at the Summer Olympics in Los Angeles, **Tessa Sanderson** won the gold medal in the women's javelin. She is the first Black woman to win gold for Great Britain and remains today the only British person to win a throwing gold medal. Tessa competed in six Olympic Games from 1976 to 1996 and has represented Great Britain for a total of 26 years, also winning three Commonwealth golds and a World Cup gold. In the March 2004 New Year's Honours list she was awarded the CBE, in recognition of her services to sport and her role as the first woman Vice Chair of Sport England. She had previously been awarded an MBE in 1985, and an OBE in 1997 for her work with various charities. Tessa's parents came to the UK as part of the Windrush generation, something she is incredibly proud of. She holds honorary degrees from South Bank University, Wolverhampton Polytechnic and a Masters from Birmingham University. She is a keynote speaker, accomplished motivational presenter and awards host, and a TV and radio personality across sport, entertainment and media. Tessa is a patron of Adoption UK and the Birmingham Commonwealth Association.

Acknowledgements

First of all, I would like to extend a huge thank-you to all of the amazing people who are the contributors to this book. You have generously shared your stories, your knowledge, your difficulties, your insights. This book is a testament to all of you. Thank you for your time, energy, patience; for working with me on your chapters, checking through edits, coming back with clarifications. I (literally) could not have done this without you and have appreciated the collaborative spirit of this book. I hope that spirit is something that comes across to readers too.

It was particularly poignant editing this book through the developing COVID-19 pandemic. The warm wishes sent and received across the globe, and the news on what was happening in your lives and your communities, have meant a great deal to me – that sense of connection during this difficult time.

Special thanks go to Dr Caroline Marfleet and to Mandu Reid, leader of the Women's Equality Party, for speaking with me for my introduction, sharing your expertise and passion.

There have been many people behind the scenes who have helped to make connections, set up interviews and spread word of the book to their contacts. I would like to thank Adela Ryle and the press office at the Women's Equality Party; Dr Bettina Pfeiderer, past chair of the Medical

Women's International Association (MWIA); Ella Simpson, Senior Lecturer in Criminology at Bath Spa University; Clean Break; Maya Campbell at Team Arzu Qaderi; Lori-Anne Sharp, Kerrie-Ann Fitzpatrick and Annie Butler at the Australian Nursing and Midwifery Federation (ANMF); Waun'Shea Blount at Johns Hopkins Medicine; Carol Bagnald at Black on Silver; Rachel Weiss and Andy Sanwell for your hospitality in Perth; and Dr Caroline Marfleet and Catherine O'Keeffe for checking parts of the text.

Also all those who have offered ideas and help with finding contributors and answered my call-outs, even if it was with a 'nice no' (kindness in our interactions with each other goes a long way).

With thanks to Bill Rukeyser for kind permission to print a quote from 'Käthe Kollwitz' by his mother Muriel Rukeyser; to Rosemarie Garland-Thomson for the quote from her chapter, 'Disability, Identity, and Representation: An Introduction', in her book *Extraordinary Bodies*; and to Lisa Robertson for the line from her *Proverbs of a She-Dandy*.

At Flint and parent company The History Press, publishing director Laura Perehinec has championed this book from the start and supported it through testing times for the publishing world. I would also like to thank Katie Beard for her striking, fitting and contemporary cover and design, and project editor Alex Waite, copyeditor Catherine Hanley and proof-reader Sarah Wright for their thoughtful attention to detail. Plus, on the marketing and promotions team, head of marketing Caitlin Kirkman, and marketing executive Molly Evans and Katie Read of Read Media, who have worked hard and creatively to make sure this book reaches a wide range of audiences. My particular and heartfelt thanks go to Jo de Vries, my commissioning editor, who has been in many ways my co-editor of this book, from shaping the initial proposal with me, to giving support and kind words when I needed them, and bringing her fine-tuned editorial judgement to the project at all of its stages.

I'd also like to acknowledge the efforts and contributions of all those involved in the chain of making and distributing this book: from its paper and printing, to shipping and warehousing, to delivery drivers, bookshops (physical and virtual), and those who share the book with others.

Finally, to Clive and Ethan, my family (along with our cat companions Oregano and the much-missed Coriander) – there are too many things to thank you for.

Menopause Literacy and Sources of Support and Information

The words we all need

Many of the people I have spoken to, and those they have spoken with, have talked about how they wished they'd had more information. Many felt they had reached menopause not knowing enough about it (and I include myself here) and wondered why they had not explored the subject themselves, or been informed in a clearly understandable way.

There are leaflets and information sources online, but we often have to seek them out for ourselves, and for many women globally these may not be available in their first language. There are calls for menopause to become part of standard curriculums, so that school students learn about it alongside puberty and child-bearing, and all doctors study it in their training. Following campaigning, the UK government announced in summer 2019 that menopause will now be part of Relationships and Sex Education (RSE), taught at secondary school.

Speaking to Mandu Reid, particularly in her role as founder of The Cup Effect, which provides education in low-income countries as well as the UK, we talked about 'menstrual literacy'. I feel strongly that 'menopause literacy' is also vitally needed.

This is partly about knowing our way around our female anatomy – both physically and experientially, so we come to understand the workings of our own bodies and can notice changes in them, and also the medical terminology, so that we can feel more confident when speaking to doctors and other healthcare professionals. It is also about knowing the stages of the menopause process and having an idea of the possible effects we might be experiencing, so we know when it could be worth pressing for a hormone level test (where these are available) or discussing possible treatments.

This 'menopause literacy' section gives some broad outlines and offers definitions of some terms used within this book. It does not go into the details of pharmaceutical treatments or 'natural' supplements, as these are best discussed on an individual basis with a qualified healthcare professional: menopause is different for each of us; we each have our own health profile, beliefs and preferences, making some options more appropriate for us than others.

Getting to know female anatomy

This is a selection of the medical terms. Chapter 18, from Dr Wen Shen and Dr Christine Ekechi, gives some very helpful explanations, too, from the perspective of women working daily in gynaecological medicine.

vagina (*vaginal*) and *vulva* (*vulval or vulvar*)
The *vagina* is the internal canal, connecting the womb to the outside. The *vulva* is all the external parts, including the 'lips' (*labia*) and *clitoris*. The *perineum* is the area between this and the anus.

uterus
The medical term for the womb. The *cervix* (as in 'cervical smear test') is the 'neck' of tissue that connects vagina and uterus. The outside of this may be felt as a mound in the vagina; its central gap or passage into the womb is called the *os* ('mouth' in Latin – still the language of so much of our 'polite' discussion about our bodies).

ovary (ovarian)
The *ovaries* are the grape-like female sex organs (or *gonads*) that contain and protect the eggs – which females are born with. They later release these eggs and also produce and secrete hormones, primarily oestrogen and progesterone. The *oviducts* (aka *fallopian tubes*) catch the eggs and conduct them towards the uterus.

female sex hormones
Hormones are chemical messengers that regulate and affect many of the processes of living, from growth to sleep, in ways there is still much to learn about. The specialist study of hormones is known as *endocrinology*. The female sex hormones are produced by the ovaries and the *adrenal glands*, at the top of each kidney (and yes, they do also produce adrenaline), as well as in other tissues. The main female sex hormones are:

oestrogen (aka O)
Plays a key role in the development of female characteristics such as breasts at puberty, in reproduction (thickening the wall of the uterus, for example) and many other areas of our health and well-being (see Chapter 18). You may hear about different types of oestrogen: oestrone, oestradiol and oestriol. (Often all spelled without the 'o', especially in the US.)

progesterone
Regulates the menstrual cycle, prepares the body for conception and is active during pregnancy, for example, helping to suppress ovulation and stimulate the growth of the milk-producing (mammary) glands.

testosterone (aka T)
Also produced by the ovaries and adrenal glands in women, and in other tissues. Female bodies generally have much lower levels than male.

Other hormones you may hear about that are relevant to menopause include *gonadotropin releasing hormone (GnRH)*, *follicle stimulating hormone (FSH)*, *luteinising hormone (LH)* and *dehydroepiandrosterone (DHEA)*.

Some conditions and procedures

adenomyosis and endometriosis

Adenomyosis is when the tissue of the uterus (*endometrial* tissue) grows into its muscle wall. It can cause an enlarged uterus and painful, heavy periods. *Endometriosis* is when tissues similar to the womb lining start growing in other places, such as the ovaries and fallopian tubes, and elsewhere in the abdomen. It can cause pain and gut distress, and have an impact on fertility.

dysphoria

Defined generally as an intense unease, unhappiness, dissatisfaction, restlessness and frustration, and recognised as a psychological state. *Gender dysphoria* is described by the NHS Gender Identity Clinic as: 'distress experienced by those whose gender identity feels at odds with aspects of their body and/or the social gender role assigned to them at birth. This can be experienced as physical discomfort, and psychological and emotional distress'.

fibroids

Benign, non-cancerous growths (tumours) in or on the uterus. There are several different types. They can cause severe pain and heavy periods for some, but few or no symptoms for others.

female sexual dysfunction (FSD)

The Hormone Health website (hormone.org) of the US Endocrine Society defines FSD as when a woman is unhappy about her sexual health. So it is about this being a problem for her, rather than a medical definition of lack. Common issues causing distress might include low libido, difficulty becoming aroused, difficulty reaching orgasm, painful sex.

hysterectomy and oophorectomy

With a *hysterectomy*, the womb is surgically removed, which can be for a number of medical reasons. An *oophorectomy* – removal of one or both ovaries – may be carried out at the same time or as a separate procedure, for example, for ovarian cancer.

premenstrual dysphoric disorder (PMDD)
Similar to PMS (premenstrual syndrome) but more severe, PMDD can bring intense depression, irritability and tension as hormone levels change in the week or more before ovulation. Research suggests it could be understood as an increased sensitivity to hormone levels (see Sophie Watkins' account in Chapter 7).

urinary tract infection (UTI)
The term for infections of the urinary system: of the bladder (*cystitis*), urethra (the tube from the bladder to outside; *urethritis*) and kidneys (kidney infection).

Menopause-related terms

menopause
What is widely referred to as 'the menopause' is a process that can take a number of years, even a decade or more. Some symptoms and effects are temporary and settle down (the 'Rockies' effect, discussed by Dr Shen). Others are progressive changes as we age beyond the ending of our periods. In medical terminology, menopause refers to the point when menstruation stops – the *final menstrual period* (FMP). You are usually counted as having gone through menopause when you have not had any periods for a year.

premenopause
The whole reproductive stage of life before menopause.

perimenopause
Medically, according to the World Health Organization and quoted by the International Menopause Society, this refers to the time immediately around menopause – just before it begins and the year afterwards. However, informally it is commonly used to refer to the longer period of time before and after menopause.

postmenopause
The time after the final menstrual period, regardless of whether this was 'natural' or induced.

early menopause
So-called 'natural' or 'spontaneous' menopause occurs for most people between the ages of 45 and 55, although the age distribution can vary in different countries. Early menopause is regarded as before 45.

premature ovarian insufficiency (POI)
POI is when menopause occurs below the age of 40 and can begin as early as teenage years. The ovaries stop producing oestrogen, progesterone and mature eggs many years before it is usual (see page 17).

medical or *induced menopause*
This refers to menopause as a result of medical treatment: both deliberately induced menopause, for example, in medical treatment for severe pain with endometriosis, and also menopause triggered by chemotherapy, radiation therapy and surgery as treatments for cancers.

hormonal induced menopause
Medical menopause induced by medications that suppress the menstrual cycle, generally as a treatment for endometriosis. Female-to-male (ftm) transitioning involves a form of hormonal menopause, although the order of treatments (as discussed by Lee Hurley in Chapter 9) is supposed to suppress menopausal symptoms.

surgical menopause
When the ovaries are removed, in an oophorectomy.

hormone replacement therapy (HRT)
Various hormones and combinations given as a medical treatment for menopause symptoms. The options available vary, for example, between different countries.

systemic HRT
Travels through the bloodstream, so potentially having an effect on the whole body (system). It may be prescribed as spray, implant, or injection.

topical HRT
Oestrogen creams, pessaries, tablets and rings to be inserted into the vagina for genitourinary syndrome of menopause (GSM) symptoms. Their effects are localised rather than systemic.

Symptoms associated with menopause

There are now more than thirty-five recognised symptoms associated with menopause, from gynaecological, to psychological and emotional, to a range of other physical symptoms and pain that can affect many areas of the body. The list was originated by Judy Bayliss and her Menopaus email support group. It is worth noting that each person's experience of menopause, and its symptoms, is likely to be different, because that experience is shaped by many factors, not only hormone levels but other aspects of our lives (see Chapter 2). You may have symptoms that do not quite fit into any of the categories here, but that does not mean you shouldn't raise them in relation to menopause – the list below is not exhaustive and doctors and researchers, like all of us, are learning more all the time. However, on the other hand, not every symptom around the time of menopause is down to hormone changes: do make sure to check with a health professional, in case there is another cause.

Some of the most common symptoms:
hot flushes and/or night sweats
irregular or very heavy periods
fatigue
inability to concentrate
mood swings
insomnia
loss of libido (and painful sex, especially intercourse, termed dyspareunia)
vaginal dryness and vulvovaginal atrophy (VVA), including thinned, frag-
    ile skin of the vagina and vulva; often grouped by doctors with bladder
    issues as genitourinary syndrome of menopause (GSM)

anxiety
irritability
depression
Mental and emotional:
brain fog
memory loss
feelings of dread, apprehension and doom (and also suicidal thoughts)
panic disorders
loss of confidence

Physical:
weight gain
bloating
gastrointestinal distress (including indigestion and nausea)
osteoporosis
brittle nails
hair loss (or hair increases, such as in pubic and facial hair)
itchy and dry skin, and other skin changes
irregular heartbeat (arrhythmia and palpitations)
allergies (and effects on other immune system-related conditions)
muscle tension
dental issues (including gum disease, or gingivitis, and bleeding)
bladder issues (urinary incontinence and urgency, and UTIs, which can become chronic; often grouped by doctors with vaginal and vulval symptoms as GSM)
changes in body odours
dizziness and loss of balance
clumsiness
tinnitus and other hearing issues

Pain-related:
joint pain
breast tenderness
headaches (including migraine)
burning mouth syndrome
tingling hands, feet and limbs (including restless leg syndrome)
electric shock sensations

Helpful books

The Vagina Bible by Dr Jen Gunter (Citadel Press, 2019)
OB-GYN doctor Jen Gunter, no-nonsense expert on women's health, debunks the myths and educates and empowers women.

Me and My Menopausal Vagina: Living With Vaginal Atrophy by Jane Lewis (PAL Books, 2018)
Honest, informative, taboo-breaking and funny account of how the author became her own expert to find what works.

The M Word: Everything You Need to Know About the Menopause by Dr Philippa Kaye (Vie, 2020)
Friendly, evidence-based and easily understandable advice on many key aspects of menopause from the GP and popular author.

Our Bodies Ourselves (first published in 1979)
Book and websites with easily understandable information on women's health. www.ourbodiesourselves.org/book-excerpts/health-topics/menopause-perimenopause/

Also see the book references from contributors for each chapter (page 299 to 303).

Organisations and support

This is by no means an entire list of the many incredible organisations that exist to offer support or advice on menopause and related conditions. We've offered a snapshot of those in the UK and some of the larger global sources, but worldwide there are a myriad of grassroots organisations that can offer rich communities of support and practical help, so do use the below as a springboard to find help closest to you.

Some of the first places you might want to start looking for support are:

Your doctor
Local hospital groups
Your workplace and unions
Mental and emotional health support networks, such as MIND

Useful factsheets

Women's Health Concern Factsheet:
www.womens-health-concern.org/help-and-advice/factsheets/
   menopause

NHS conditions: Menopause:
www.nhs.uk/conditions/menopause

NICE guidelines for diagnosis and treatment of menopause:
www.nice.org.uk/guidance/qs143

Australasian Menopause Society Fact Sheets:
www.menopause.org.au/health-info/fact-sheets

International Menopause Society Fact Sheet:
www.imsociety.org/downloads/world_menopause_day_2011/wmd_
   general_menopause_backgrounder.pdf

BDA Fact Sheet about Menopause and Diet:
www.bda.uk.com/resource/menopause-diet.html

Organisations in the UK

The British Menopause Society
The British Menopause Society (BMS), established in 1989, educates, informs and guides healthcare professionals in all aspects of post-reproductive health. It offers a range of publications, including quarterly journal *Post Reproductive Health* and the handbook *Management of the Menopause*.
thebms.org.uk

Menopause Support
Run by menopause campaigner Diane Danzebrink, who is a professional coach, counsellor and trauma therapist with nurse training in the menopause (see Chapter 3). She is the media lay spokesperson for the Royal College of Obstetricians and Gynaecologists, a member of the RCOG Women's Voices Involvement Panel and a member of the British Menopause Society.
menopausesupport.co.uk

Henpicked
An organisation of menopause in the workplace experts, who provide line manager and colleague training, videos, e-learning, policy and communications expertise.
menopauseintheworkplace.co.uk

Ovacome
Ovacome is the national UK ovarian cancer charity focused on providing support to anyone affected by ovarian cancer, and can offer support to those affected by surgical menopause due to these conditions.
www.ovacome.org.uk

Endometriosis UK
Endometriosis UK works to improve the lives of people affected by endometriosis and to decrease the impact it has on those with the condition and their families and friends.
www.endometriosis-uk.org/get-support

Menopause Café®
At a Menopause Café people, often strangers, gather to eat cake, drink tea and discuss menopause (see Chapter 20). Menopause Cafés are also starting up in workplaces and around the world.
www.menopausecafe.net

Global organisations

The Daisy Network
The Daisy Network supports those experiencing premature menopause, premature ovarian failure and/or premature ovarian insufficiency (POI).
www.daisynetwork.org

International Menopause Society (IMS) and local branches
The IMS works to promote and support access to best-practice healthcare for women through menopause and beyond. It has national and regional affiliates such as the British Menopause Society, North American Menopause Society (US and Canada) and organisations from Asia Pacific to Nicaragua, South Africa to the United Arab Emirates.
www.imsociety.org

Medical Women's International Association (MWIA)
A global organisation of women working in medicine.
mwia.net/

Endometriosis.org
Delivers up-to-date, evidence-based information and news about
endometriosis, to provide the knowledge that empowers women to make
informed decisions about their treatment options.
endometriosis.org/

Websites and forums

An online search will turn up a growing number of blogs, magazine-style
websites and forums around the world.

My Second Spring
Aisling Grimley's site was one of the first dedicated to menopause, with an
active online community across the globe.
mysecondspring.ie/

Menopaus
Menopaus is an email support group for and about women who believe
they are experiencing the effects of perimenopause, menopause or post
menopause.
menopaus.icors.org/menolist.htm

Menopause Matters
An award-winning, independent website providing up-to-date, accurate
information about the menopause, menopausal symptoms and treatment
options. Here you will find information on what happens leading up to,
during and after the menopause, what the consequences can be, what you
can do to help and what treatments are available.
www.menopausematters.co.uk/

Gender GP
GenderGP is a worldwide online health and well-being service offering HRT,
support, counselling, medication, monitoring and advice to transgender
people.
www.gendergp.com/

Annual events

World Menopause Day
Takes place annually on 18 October, and the World Health Organization has designated October as World Menopause Month.

The M Word Event
Annual event in Ireland exploring menopause topics and providing an empowering, educated day with experts.

#FlushFest
The Menopause Festival in Perth, Scotland, with information, menopause at work, and celebrations.

MegsMenopause® Conference
An annual medical conference, organised by menopause campaigner Meg Mathews.

Sources used throughout the book

Introduction

Charlap, C. (2019, rev. ed.) *La Fabrique de la Ménopause* (*The Construction of the Menopause*), Paris: CNRS Editions

Criado Perez, C. (2019) *Invisible Women: Exposing Data Bias in a World Designed for Men*, London: Chatto & Windus

Government Equalities Office and the Rt Hon Justine Greening (2017) 'Menopause Transition: Effects on Women's Economic Participation', Gov.uk

Hagège, S. (February 2020) 'Is Menopause a Social Construct?: An Interview with Cécile Charlap', CNRS News

Jackson, G. (2019) *Pain and Prejudice: A Call to Arms for Women and Their Bodies*, London: Little, Brown

Sheehy, G. (October 1991) 'The Silent Passage: Menopause', *Vanity Fair*

Sheehy, G. (1992) *The Silent Passage*, New York: Random House

Chapter 1

Anderson, G. and Nadel, J. (2017) *WE: A Manifesto for Women Everywhere*, London: Harper Thornson

Chapter 2

Bahri N., and Latifnejad, R. (2015) 'Menopause Research Studies through Passage of Time: Shifting from Biomedical to Holistic Approaches', *Iranian Journal of Obstetrics, Gynecology and Infertility*, 18(154):19–34

British Menopause Society (October 2017) 'Fact Sheet: A Woman's Relationship with the Menopause Is Complicated'

Chen, Y.L., Voda, A.M., Mansfield, P.K. (1998) 'Chinese Midlife Women's Perceptions and Attitudes about Menopause', *Menopause*, 5:28–34

Cheng, M.H., Wang, S.J., Wang, P.H., Fuh, J.L. (2005) 'Attitudes Toward Menopause Among Middle-aged Women: A Community Survey in an Island of Taiwan', *Maturitas*, 52:348–355

Dennerstein, L., Smith, A.M., Morse, C. (1994) 'Psychological Well-being, Mid-life and the Menopause', *Maturitas*, 20:1–11

E.ON. (18 October 2017) 'E.ON becomes Britain's First Menopause-friendly Energy Company'

Harel, C.M. (22 January 2020) 'Hollywood's Menopause Problem: The Silence Around It Perpetuates Silence Among Women', *The Hollywood Reporter*

Hassan, A. (20 March 2019) 'Menopausal Women Aren't Being Supported at Work—and It's Affecting Companies' Bottom Line', Quartz

Health Line (21 March 2019) 'The Best Menopause Blogs of 2019', Health Line

Hope, C. (21 July 2017) 'Menopause Costs Economy Millions Every Year because Bosses Do Not Understand It, Government Says', *The Telegraph*

Hunter, M.S. (1990) 'Psychological and Somatic Experience of the Menopause: A Prospective Study', *Psychosomatic Medicine*, 52:357–367

Lee, M-S, Kim, J-H, Park, M.S., *et al.* (2010) 'Factors Influencing the Severity of Menopause Symptoms in Korean Post-Menopausal Women', *Journal of Korean Medical Science*, 25(5):758–765. doi:10.3346/jkms.2010.25.5.758

Lock, M. (May–August 1994) 'Menopause in Cultural Context', *Experimental Gerontology*; 29(3–4): 307–317

Namazi, M., *et al.* (2019) 'Social Determinants of Health in Menopause: An Integrative Review', *International Journal of Women's Health*, 11: 637–647

Rappaport, L. (June 2015) 'Culture May Influence How Women Experience Menopause', Reuters

Sharan, T. (2017) 'The Menopause Mantra: Learn How to Enjoy a New Beginning', *The Better India*

Shariat, S., and Simbar, M. (2014) 'Relationship of Perceived Social Support with Women's Experiences in Menopause', *Advances in Nursing & Midwifery*, 25(90)

University of Leicester (11 May 2018) 'University of Leicester Menopause Policy'

U.S. Bureau of Labor Statistics (December 2015) 'U.S. Bureau of Labor Statistics Labor Force Projections to 2024: The Labor Force is Growing, but Slowly'

Chapter 4

Huston, J.E., Lanka, L.D. and Jovanovic, L. (2001) *Perimenopause: Changes in Women's Health After 35*, California: New Harbinger Publications

Rediker, M. (2007) *The Slave Ship: A Human History*, New York: Viking

Chapter 8

Strock, C. (2008) *Married Women Who Love Women*, New York: Routledge

Chapter 10

Cox, J., and Sacks-Jones, K. (April 2017) '"Double disadvantage" The experiences of Black, Asian and Minority Ethnic women in the criminal justice system', Agenda, the alliance for women and girls at risk, and Women in Prison (WIP)

Escobar, N., and Plugge, E. (23 October 2019) 'Prevalence of human papillomavirus infection, cervical intraepithelial neoplasia and cervical cancer in imprisoned women worldwide: a systematic review and meta-analysis', *Journal of Epidemiology and Community Health* 2020, 74:95–102

HM Prison & Probation Service, *The Prison Service Instructions*

Jewkes, Y., *et al.* (2007) *Handbook on Prisons*, Abingdon: Routledge

Lammy, D. (September 2017) 'The Lammy Review'

London, B., Downey, G., Romero-Canyas, R., Rattan, A., and Tyson, D. (2012) 'Gender-based rejection sensitivity and academic self-silencing in women', *Journal of Personality and Social Psychology*, 102(5):961–979

Peden, J., and McCann, L., *et al.* (2018) 'Gender Specific Standards to Improve Health and Well-being for Women in Prison in England', Public Health England

Prison Reform Trust (2008) 'Doing Time: The Experiences and Needs of Older People in Prison', London: Prison Reform Trust

National Audit Office (9 March 2006) 'Serving Time: Prisoner Diet and Exercise', London: The Stationery Office

Chapter 11

Garland-Thomson, R., 'Disability, Identity, and Representation: An Introduction' in *Extraordinary Bodies*, New York: Columbia University Press

Robertson, L. (2017) *Proverbs of a She-Dandy*, Vancouver, BC: Morris and Helen Belkin Art Gallery

Rukeyser, M. 'Käthe Kollwitz', Poetry Foundation, www.poetryfoundation.org/poems/90874/kathe-kollwitz

Chapter 12

Rosenhek, J. (February 2014) 'Mad with Menopause: The way we look at The Change has certainly, well, changed', *Doctor's Review*

Chapter 13

Mosconi, L. (2020) *The XX Brain: The Groundbreaking Science Empowering Women to Prevent Dementia*, Crow's Nest: Allen & Unwin

Chapter 15

Bourland, B. (3 August 2017) 'Stop trying to be beautiful', *Grazia*

Fredrickson, B., Roberts, T.A., Noll, S.M., Quinne, D.M., and Twenge, J.M. (1998) 'That swimsuit becomes you: Sex differences in self-objecti-fication, restrained eating, and math performance', *Journal of Personality and Social Psychology*, 75(1):269–284

Gadsden, L.H. (6 November 2018) 'The troubling news about black women in the workplace', *Forbes*

Girl Guiding (2014) *Girl's Attitudes Survey 2014*

Korn Ferry (4 March 2016) *Women are better at using soft skills crucial for effective leadership and superior business performance finds Korn Ferry*

Miles, R. (1989) *The Women's History of the World*, London: Palladin Books

Onley, D. (3 March 2019) 'U.S. Circuit Court rules it is legal to refuse jobs to people with dreadlocks' *The Grio*

Rippon, G. (2019) *The Gendered Brain*, London: Penguin Random House

Walker, B.G. (1985) *The Crone: Woman of Age Wisdom and Power*, San Francisco: Harper and Row Publishers

Chapter 16

Ussher, J., Hawkey, A. and Perz. J. (2019) '"Age of Despair", or "When Life Starts": Migrant and Refugee Women Negotiate Constructions of Menopause', *Culture Health and Sexuality*, 21(7):741–756

Suad, J. ed. (2005) *Encyclopedia of Women and Islamic Cultures vol. 3: Family, Body, Sexuality and Health*, Brill

Chapter 18
Ekechi, Dr C. (May 2019) 'BAME women are let down by the health system – nowhere more so than in gynaecological health', Inews

Chapter 19
Franks, L. (2005) *The SEED Handbook: The Feminine Way to Create Business*, California: Hay House

Chapter 20
Fong, J. (2017) *The Death Café Movement: Exploring the Horizons of Mortality*, London: Palgrave Macmillan

Oldenburg, R. (2001) *Celebrating the Third Place: Inspiring Stories About the Great Good Places at the Heart of Our Communities*, Cambridge, Mass.: Da Capo Press

Rohr, R. (2012) *Falling Upward: A Spirituality for the Two Halves of Life*, London: SPCK Publishing

♀